Critical Voices in Child and Adolescent Mental Health

Edited by:

Sami Timimi and Begum Maitra

Published in the United Kingdom 2005
by Free Association Books
London

© Free Association Books 2005

British Library Cataloguing in Publication Data
A catalogue record for this book is available from the British Library

Produced by Bookchase, London
Printed and bound in the EU

ISBN 1853439436

Contents

About the authors

EIA ASEN, is both a Consultant Child and Adolescent Psychiatrist and a Consultant Psychiatrist in Psychotherapy. He is the clinical director of the Marlborough Family Service, which is a publicly funded (NHS) integrated Child and Adolescent Mental Health Service and Adult Psychotherapy service in Central London. He has received psychodynamic training and also trained as a family and couple therapist. He is the author and co-author of 7 books, as well as many scientific papers and book chapters. He lectures all over Europe and has been involved in a number of research projects, on depression, eating disorders, family violence and educational failure.

RAJEEV GOPAL BANHATTI, is a consultant child and adolescent psychiatrist in Northampton. UK. He trained in Pune, India as a general psychiatrist and continued further training in the UK in child psychiatry. He lives with wife Seema and two children, Ruchi and Suhrud. Marathi, English and Hindi are the languages used (in that order) at home. His interest in Indian culture and philosophy has been rekindled of late and he has been especially interested in Attention Deficit Hyperactivity Disorder, attachment and culture in general for many years. He is a visiting lecturer to University College Northampton. His hobbies include travel, reading and listening to many types of music.

KEDAR NATH DWIVEDI, (formerly Consultant Child Psychiatrist) is the Director of International Institute of Child and Adolescent Mental Health and Course Director of Midland Course in Group work with Children and Adolescents. He has edited/co-edited books on 'Group Work with Children and Adolescents' (Jessica Kingsley), 'Enhancing Parenting Skills' (Wiley), 'Therapeutic Use of Stories' (Routledge), 'Meeting the Needs of Ethnic Minority Children' (Jessica Kingsley), 'Promoting Emotional Well Being of Children and Adolescents' (Jessica Kingsley), 'Depression in Children and Adolescents' (Whurr), 'Handbook of Childhood Anxiety Disorders' (Ashgate) and 'Posttraumatic Stress Disorder in Children and Adolescents' (Whurr).

JON JUREIDINI, Child Psychiatrist, is head, Department of Psychological Medicine, Women's and Children's Hospital, Adelaide, where he is also on the patient care ethics committee. He is Senior Research Fellow, Department of Philosophy, Flinders University and is a Clinical Senior Lecturer in the Department of Psychiatry, University of Adelaide. He is the Chair of Healthy Skepticism (www.healthyskepticism.org). Publications in the last 2 years have addressed immigration detention, parenting, prescribing for children, narrative, dissociation and consciousness, placebo analgesia, child abuse, and rehabilitation of adolescents with unexplained symptoms.

JONATHAN LEO, is an associate professor of anatomy at Lake Erie College of Osteopathic Medicine in Bradenton Florida, where he teaches gross anatomy and neuroscience to medical students. He has written several articles about the oversimplification of the biological theories of mental illness so often found in professional and lay publications. 'The Biology of Mental Illness' was recently published in *Society*, and 'Broken Brains or Flawed Studies: A Critical Review of ADHD Neuroimaging Research', co-authored with David Cohen, appeared in *The Journal of Mind and Behavior*. He is the co-editor-in-chief of the journal, *Ethical Human Psychology and Psychiatry*.

BEGUM MAITRA, Consultant Child and Adolescent Psychiatrist, East London and The City Mental Health NHS Trust, and Jungian Analyst. Her interest in the subject of cultural psychiatry began with her initial psychiatric training in India, and has developed to include the impact of culture on children, families and on the practice of mental health. Dr Maitra has a keen interest in research within this area, and has been consultant to research studies of national relevance on minority ethnic children and families within child care proceedings. She has published on assessment of parenting across cultures in cases of child abuse/neglect, on cultural therapy and cultural competence and training.

PETER R MANSFIELD, is an Australian GP and founder of Healthy Skepticism, an international organisation aiming to reducing harm from misleading drug promotion. Peter designed the organisation (originally the Medical Lobby for Appropriate Marketing) by merging ideas from every inhabited continent during his final year student elective in Bangladesh in 1982. In 2003, Peter was awarded a Centenary Medal by the Australian Government 'for contributions to Australian society especially through Healthy Skepticism' and a Convocation Medal by Flinders University for 'outstanding leadership in the advancement of professional practice and service to the community in the safe use of pharmaceutical drugs'.

ELISSE MOODY, qualified as a Registered Mental Nurse in 1984 and for the first few years worked within adult acute psychiatry, elderly services and adult community services. In 1998 she joined the Child and Adolescent Mental Health Service community team and worked as a liaison nurse specialist for 4 years, completing the Diploma in Child, Adolescent and Family Mental Health and the foundation year in Systemic Family Therapy. She then became Unit and Project Manager for the in-patient adolescent unit in Lincolnshire. She is a mother to four teenage daughters.

SAMI TIMIMI, is a consultant child and adolescent psychiatrist who works full time in the NHS in Lincolnshire, as consultant to the county adolescent in-patient unit and to a community service. In addition to general psychiatry and child psychiatry training he has also trained in psychodynamic psychotherapy, group psychotherapy, family therapy and hypnotherapy. He has published many papers in peer-reviewed journals on a variety of topics including eating disorders, psychotherapy, ADHD, depression and cross-cultural psychiatry. He has published two books '*Pathological Child Psychiatry and the Medicalization of Childhood*' in 2002, and '*Naughty Boys: Anti-social behaviour, ADHD and the Role of Culture*' in 2005.

CHARLES L. WHITFIELD, is a pioneer in trauma recovery, including the way we remember childhood and other trauma and abuse. He is the author of fifty published articles and six best selling books on trauma psychology and recovery, three of these books have been translated and published in ten foreign languages. For over twenty-three years he has taught at Rutgers University's Institute on Alcohol and Drug Studies. He has been a consultant and research collaborator at the CDC since 1998. He has a private practice in Atlanta, where he provides individual and group therapy for trauma survivors and people with addictions and other problems in living.

DAVID WOODHOUSE, trained as a P.E. and Maths teacher in England and taught for a number of years in secondary schools prior to undertaking his post-graduate studies at the University of North Carolina. He taught at the University of North Carolina and then worked in a Centre for Integrated Education at the University of South Carolina before returning to England. For the past twenty-five years he has been teaching and researching in higher education institutions in England. He was the Head of Psychology at the University of Teesside for ten years and became the Director of the Cactus Clinic, which is based at the University, following the death of Professor Steve Baldwin who founded the clinic.

Preface

T he idea for this book arose out of the knowledge that other writers and professionals, also in the field of child and adolescent mental health for a long time, were critiquing mainstream ideology and current practice, and were looking outside these areas to try and develop new ways of thinking and practicing. We know of many clinicians who are as concerned as we are about the direction child and adolescent mental health has been heading, and especially about the impact of the biomedical 'colonisation' of the institutions we work within and ultimately on the children and families who seek our help. Not everyone who shares our concerns wants to write about it. Verbalising one's criticisms of mainstream practice exposes one to the power of the 'old guard', and its effect in marginalizing dissenting voices. This can make for a lonely and threatened professional existence. One of our reasons for attempting to pull together a variety of critical voices, new ideas and new thinking in a book like this is to resist this isolation, and to point to a community of professionals and academics who, like us, are trying to widen the boundaries of professional thinking and practice around children's mental health.

In planning this book we approached a number of clinicians considered 'outside the mainstream', some of whom had already published and whose work we knew to be innovative. Not all the authors we approached were able to contribute this book. Those who have contributed have a wide range of interests, and adopt a range of positions with regard to their relation to mainstream thinking and practice, whether to mount a radical critique of it, or to suggest approaches that modify or 'complement' it. Our interest in the diversity of existing opinions meant that we did not expect to agree with the content of all the chapters, but we did wish to urge authors to clarify their positions on these debates. While we might have wished for a more radical critique of current thinking in certain areas, some authors decided not to pick up on our ideas and suggestions in response to their first drafts. With others, such as in the chapter on Indian childhoods we (BM) have joined them, hoping to emphasise that any one account of a culture cannot hope to speak for the diversity of views held by all its members, or to claim that it represents a more truthful 'historical' account than that of another. This seems particularly important in a period such as ours in which claims for 'authentic', singular truths must be viewed with a healthy scepticism. This unevenness does not seem problematic to us. It was not our intention to write a 'homogenous' book.

The point of this book is to give voice to ideas that are currently marginal, that we think have something interesting to say, either about theory or practice. We feel the richness of this book lies in its not privileging consensus over debate. We also believe that there is no given end point to any critique and thus we don't see any of the chapters in this book as making 'final' statements about the subjects under discussion. What we would like to see are critiques and new ideas, like those in this book, helping to provide new opportunities for us to take risks and ask the sorts of questions that may spur new research and new ways of exploring the subject matter. What we would like to see in child and adolescent mental health is theory and practice that is in constant dialogue, not only within its own members, but also with other disciplines, and with its clients. What we believe must change is the view that our current knowledge base in child and adolescent mental health, represents a concrete body of truth that can be applied universally to all children and that is handed down from one generation to the next. We hope this book can contribute to this process.

We are aware of how easy it is for positions to become polarised in any such debate. Those who believe that current thinking is based on 'fact' may see critiques of it as angry and destructive acts. While it is true that these are not dispassionate critiques, for how could any opposition to the 'institutionalised racism' within the National Health Service (Coker, 2001) and the academic bodies that train mental health professionals remain so. Several of the authors in this volume, including ourselves, have personal and professional experience of coherent and functional beliefs and practices around children, framed within very different cultural systems than those that continue to dominate Western trainings and practise. This persistent blindness to diversity is not merely 'academic' but wrings a significant cost in 'misdiagnosis', non-attendance, failure of service provision (sometimes glossed over as 'non-compliance') for the public it claims to serve (Maitra, 2004), and in failing to deliver a highly skilled service that is alert to changing needs. It is not surprising either that the persistent failure to acknowledge and utilise the skills of bi-cultural (especially non-Western) professionals, particularly in the context of constant cries of 'stretched resources' in a 'First World' state, creates a situation of conflict between professionals who would maintain the status quo and those who press for a re-evaluation of our knowledge base and our practices. This poses a difficult challenge and delicate balancing act for us, and is not merely a wish to retaliate or to subvert the current power base. While many return to their countries, sometimes defeated by the complexities of trying to influence the evolution of ideas, others such as ourselves have remained working in Britain, and have found ways of bringing the richness of our experiences, both professional and personal, into our work with British and other cultural groups. We have persisted in the belief that we could bring to theory and practice something new, interesting and hopefully constructive. This book is another means to promote more open consideration of the voices, research and publications that have 'traditionally' been marginalized by the academic disciplines that contribute to policy and practice in child and family mental health. We believe that such openness is the only possible route to robust new ideas, and to a more direct relationship between policy makers, practitioners and service users. This book hopes to contribute by bringing the ideas expressed in it into the mainstream.

It is important, in trying to neutralize the fear of what is new and unconventional, not to misrepresent those who genuinely believe in the premises that current Western theory and practice are based on. We believe that our colleagues are more often than not genuinely concerned with trying to do the best for their patients, and that the problem lies not with individual practitioners so much as with the institutionalization of theory and practice to the point where it ceases to examine its own premises, and fails to see when these have been ruled obsolete by changing society and public need. Such institutionalized rigidity within academic bodies inevitably has a powerful influence on how alternative points of view are treated, whether these are treated with suspicion, dismissed without examination, or welcomed as material from which new ideas might arise.

Part of these institutionalized biases, we think, results from the institutionalized racism that lies at the heart of the conceptual systems we use in psychiatry. This is of course a painful issue for doctors to face, as a thorough examination of our guiding institutional philosophies could lead to our profession being diagnosed as being deeply disturbed (just as the UK police were with the Stephen Lawrence enquiry). Such an analysis would reveal that the core assumptions of the theory base, and consequently of practice, in psychiatry, developed during an era where racism was the accepted norm, and where the intellectual and psychological superiority of the European over the colonized 'primitive' was not questioned. We should not be surprised that there are inherently racist concepts embedded in our institutionalized ways of thinking about mental health problems, how to conceptualise them, what to do about them, and in the value systems we unquestioningly take into daily practice. Mental health ideology and 'technology' developed not as the result of the discovery of testable physical pathology, but through a system of consensus (sometimes initiated by a single influential individual – Carey, 2005) among powerful psychiatrists about the significance of certain phenomena selected from the wide variety of observations that constituted the existing evidence at that time. From the beginnings of the current diagnostic systems used in psychiatry, influential psychiatrists have generally been white Western males and naturally carried their own cultural assumptions, from which a system thinking and acting for psychiatrists was developed. Our intention, in making reference to the cultural, gender and class bias of current theory and practice, is not to dismiss it all as discriminatory, but to point to the need to for its re-evaluation, and to be more explicit about what was local, and context-bound, and what might be thought of as 'universal'.

As we try to juggle this balancing act between influencing the mainstream while knowing that we are at times angry at the restrictiveness of the marginal position, it is inevitable that this will sometimes lead to conflicts with our colleagues. Sometimes the first step to influencing the powerful is through conflict. Sometimes you need to rock the boat a little to introduce something new to the system (a strategy often used in family therapy). After all when 'difference' is introduced, thinking has to happen, creativity develops and new possibilities start to emerge.

There have been many movements critical of psychiatry in the past. Movements similarly critical of child and adolescent psychiatry are relatively young, probably because the profession is relatively young. However, we need to learn from the mistakes of past critical movements, as many did not succeed in influencing mainstream practice. In recent years UK Critical Psychiatry Network (of which we are both members) has been trying to do just that. The Critical Psychiatry Network has for many years now been trying to influence psychiatric practice in the UK through publications (in mainstream peer reviewed journals), conferences, and campaigning, in an attempt to engage the profession in a constructive dialogue and debate and gain greater recognition for the importance of cross-disciplinary perspectives, a more thorough engagement with users and a move away from a focus on the technical aspects of our work and toward the ethical. Their aim, like ours, is to get more mainstream recognition for theory and practice founded on such approaches.

That theory and practice in our field should stand still and avoid engagement with wider political, cultural, and social circumstances is not acceptable. Children's lives and environments are constantly changing, often unpredictably and in ways that are hard to identify and interpret. In order to remain relevant to children's lives, child and adolescent mental health theory and practice needs a robust capacity for self-reflection and self-critique, and a willingness to incorporate new ideas and new practices. Continuing population movements due to economic reasons, wars or natural catastrophe, and the global exchange of ideas and products also mean that definitions of the 'well-being' of children will continue to be modified. If our best ideas about normal and abnormal function continue to be defined by theories of 'stable' family life based on a picture of two parents, two children, a dog, and a Ford Mondeo, then we might as well give up!

There are, we believe, reasons for some optimism. We are aware that what is considered mainstream changes over time, and that the 'centre' is constantly influenced by what lies in the margins. The loosening of all sorts of boundaries ushered in by the forces of globalisation will continue to reinforce ideas about heterogeneity and multiplicity, ensuring that 'common' culture encompasses a great diversity of views, sources and intentions. We can see that, for example, in the way political pressures change over time resulting in institutional changes. This can be seen in the wider economics of the National Health Service (NHS) in the UK, in changes in how it is funded and staffed. The current push to recruit overseas doctors, and the increasing proportion of minority ethnic medical students and trainee doctors, creates the possibility, however unintentional, for new voices to be heard. Whilst political intentions bear a complex relationship with the 'needs' of the public (one recent and worrying outcome is evident in the drive to allocate a greater policing role to psychiatrists) one of the interesting developments has been the promotion of a more user-friendly NHS (in rhetoric at least), with some effort being made to increase the involvement and influence of user organisations.

We are also encouraged by some of the leading medical journals, particularly the British Medical Journal (BMJ), which has shown an active interest in examining the premises and authority of biomedicine, and in engaging in a dialogue with other disciplines. For example, in recent years the BMJ has published a special issue devoted to the influence of the pharmaceutical industry and the medicalisation of dissatisfaction, on new models of chronic illness incorporating a greater social dimension, the social construction of sexuality, and on 'post-psychiatry' to name but a few. Indeed a shortened version of one of the chapters in this book appeared in the BMJ in December 2004 (Timimi, 2004).

We are also aware of an interesting paradox we may find ourselves in, should some of the ideas contained in this book become 'mainstream'. These ideas, like any others, are just as likely to become rigid, losing their radical edge and deteriorating into 'dogma'. Now in the 'senior' layer of our professions and no longer at risk of being dismissed as 'young radicals' (though open to being considered as 'dementing' dead wood!) it remains as urgent as ever to ensure that our institutions value and promote self-criticism and a sense of being accountable to the public with whom, as practitioners rather than theoreticians alone, we bear a close and mutually dependent relationship. We would then be able to look forward to the next generation of radical critics and to hope that they will continue to bring that sense of vitality that comes with active challenge and debate.

So what we hope this book encourages is debate, constructive critique, risk taking, an attitude of questioning and an enthusiasm for dialogue particularly in those entering the field. We hope these ideas find their way into child mental health trainings and that trainees are encouraged to develop the faculty for reflective thinking, and to think outside of the current narrow epistemology. We would like to see debate, and consequently theory and practice move beyond its current emphasis on consensus (leading more reliably to mediocrity than innovation) into something more rigorous and thoughtful. We fear that without such debate our profession (child and adolescent psychiatry) risks losing its credibility due to its failure to engage with the changing circumstances of our population. This will make it less likely that we will contribute to how families' and children's lives are shaped, and will increase the risk of the profession being used increasingly to police them on behalf of the state and society, through the wielding of the prescription pad. Let us hope we start to look outside our own branch on the tree of knowledge and start to see the rest of the tree.

Sami Timimi and Begum Maitra
February 2005

References

Carey, B. (2005) *Snake Phobias, Moodiness and A Battle in Psychiatry.* The New York Times, June 14, 2005.

Coker, N. (ed) (2001) *Racism In Medicine – An Agenda for Change.* London: Kings Fund.

Maitra, B. (2004) Would cultural matching ensure culturally competent assessments? In (Eds) P. Reder, S. Duncan and C. Lucey – *Studies in the Assessment of Parenting.* London: Routledge.

Timimi, S. (2004) *Rethinking Childhood Depression.* British Medical Journal 329, 1394-1396.

1
Introduction

Sami Timimi · Begum Maitra

Child and adolescent mental health theory and practice have come to be dominated by a psychiatric biomedical frame which is reflected in the rising numbers of children being diagnosed with 'psychiatric' illnesses and being given psychotropic medication to 'treat' these supposed diseases. This book brings together a number of authors from a variety of countries, who share a deep concern about the direction mainstream theory and practice has been heading over the past decade. These 'critical voices' draw on research and writing from related disciplines (that are rarely taken seriously in mainstream child and adolescent psychiatry) such as sociology, cultural studies, critical psychology, politics, psychotherapy, orthomolecular psychiatry, anthropology and philosophy in order to offer new ways of thinking about theory and of helping users of our services. Radical questioning of a discipline's most cherished assumptions has a long and important history in adult mental health; we see books such as this one as first steps into developing similarly critical voices from within child and adolescent mental health.

The culture of child and adolescent mental health

How do we decide that a child has a 'mental illness' or 'psychiatric disorder', or that she has in some way deviated from our notions of 'health'? How do we work out what normal, 'healthy' child development is, and which child rearing approaches contribute to these healthy outcomes? We suggest that any contemporary attempt to address these questions requires that we place culture at the heart of our thinking. It remains unclear how much of health, (especially when considering children and 'mental' health), may be considered to be independent of culture since the very process of giving meaning to behaviours and events is shaped by the cultural contexts we live in. Culture has been defined in many ways. Clarke et al (1975: 10) write of it as the ". . . *peculiar and distinctive way of life of a group, the meanings, values and ideas embodied in institutions, in social relations, in systems of belief, in customs, in the uses of objects and material life. . . the 'maps of meaning' that make things intelligible to its members*". It is common to examine, analyse and think about how systems of beliefs, customs and maps of meaning affect the attitudes and practices of other populations. The same must apply to us; making it necessary that we examine the impact our own cultures have on us, both in our personal lives and as child mental health professionals.

Western child psychiatric cultures have their roots in the European enlightenment, and a range of cultural ideas arising from, or supported by it. These include the preoccupation with the individual subject, with reason and the distinctions between the mental and physical realms. The concern with reason has led to a belief that a framework of health and illness derived from medical science is the best way to engage with mental phenomena. Thus, psychiatry sought to replace spiritual, moral, political and folk ideas of the disturbances in behaviour and mental function (commonly termed 'madness') with the framework of neuroscience and 'psycho'-pathology. The preoccupation with the individual led to a focus on his mental functions, locating madness internally, and separating it from background context. The promise to control madness through medical science has placed the psychiatric profession in an ideal situation to be both influenced by, and to influence, the politics of social exclusion, allocating to psychiatrists the power and responsibility of agents of social control (Bracken and Thomas, 2001). Child mental health services trace a more mixed lineage than that of Western bio-medicine, drawing from the fields of education, social work, psychoanalysis and systemic thinking to name a few. An awareness of the cultural roots of our professions would facilitate greater alertness to the models of health that we choose to guide our practice, as well as promote understanding of the impact of our models on the beliefs and practices of the culture we practise in.

Durkheim (1925) believed a society could neither create nor recreate itself without at the same time creating an ideal. To decide that certain behaviours on the part of our children are deviant requires a value judgment. What a society then judges as good or bad for its children depends on what it intends to make of them, and the model to which it wants them to conform. Thus Robert Colts (1986) argues that as children grow into the value system of any given culture, they are absorbed and moulded by that culture's vision of what they should become. As a result a nation's politics becomes the child's everyday psychology.

Current practice in child psychiatry shows a phenomenal increase in prescriptions of psychotropic medication to children and adolescents in most Western countries (Pincus et al, 1998; Olfson et al, 2002; Wong et al, 2004). This reflects changes in our conceptualisation of the mental health of children, and that our beliefs about what constitute the boundaries of a 'normal' child-hood have narrowed (Timimi, 2002; 2004; 2005). Our changing constructions of childhood imply that the meanings we give to children's behaviour even within the same culture or society change over time (and are likely to continue to do so). This makes suspect the idea that we know what a 'universal' normal childhood is. Given the political and economic influence of Western states, there is a danger that ideas and practices we construct in the West are inappropriately exported worldwide. A critical approach to evaluating our professional practice requires us to consider the impact of our work, not only on the clients we see, but also on the wider culture, both nearby and distant.

Whilst these important contextual issues are beginning to receive attention in adult psychiatry, the debate on how such dynamics have affected child psychiatric practice is in its infancy (Timimi, 2002). For example, the element of social control in the rising use of psychotropic medications for the behavioural control of children is only recently receiving some attention in mainstream journals (e.g. Timimi and Taylor, 2004; Timimi, 2004).

The social construction of childhood:

Whilst the immaturity of children is a biological fact, the ways in which this immaturity is understood and made meaningful is a fact of culture (Prout and James, 1997). Members of any culture hold a working definition of childhood, its nature, limitations and duration based on a network of ideas that link children with other members and with the social ecology (Harkness and Super, 1996). While they may not explicitly discuss this definition, write about it, or even consciously conceive of it as an issue, they act upon these assumptions in all of their dealings with, fears for, and expectations of, their children (Calvert, 1992). Our ideas about what makes a normal/pathological childhood are not 'innocent' of current political, economic, moral or indeed health concerns. Rather childhood often represents a central arena through which we construct our fantasies about the future and a battleground through which we struggle to express competing ideological agendas. This means that a culture's definition of normal/deviant childhoods varies not only between cultures but also within cultures over time, requiring us to explore how concepts of normal/deviant childhood and child rearing have changed over time in any given culture (vertical evidence) and between cultures (horizontal evidence).

Western childhoods

Western notions of childhood can be traced to the late seventeenth century when Locke published his influential *Some Thoughts Concerning Education.* Locke proposed that children should be viewed as individuals waiting to be moulded into shape by adults. In the mid-eighteenth century, Rousseau, in the equally influential *Emile,* argued that children were born with innate goodness that could be corrupted by certain kinds of education. These two books were crucial in paving the way for a new focus in European culture on childhood, which was now being viewed as requiring separate needs/expectations than adulthood. By the mid-nineteenth century, childhood was viewed as a distinct entity requiring protection and fostering through school education. Using the perceived social crisis of the time, the ruling classes used these new values to paint working class children as the source of many social problems, and as children who, as a result of being neglected by their parents, were a potential danger to society as future juvenile delinquents and criminals. This helped smooth the way for mass education and helped prepare public opinion for introducing the state into the parent/child relationship (Hendrick, 1997).

By the beginning of the twentieth century children in Western, capitalist states were seen as individuals on whom the state could have a more fundamental influence than their families. Now that children were all in schools they also became readily available to a variety of professionals for all sorts of 'scientific' surveys. Professional interest in the idea of child development grew and the scientific study of the individual child was encouraged in an effort to produce 'guiding principles' to be offered to parents and teachers. The medical and psychological professions helped popularize the view that childhood is marked by stages in normal development. A number of assumptions derived from psycho-medicine about what constituted normal childhood development and normal parenting were made. At the same time the state was becoming more interventionist through legislation following a debate about children's rights and an assumption that only the state could enforce these rights (Hendrick, 1997).

Before the onset of the Second World War, Western society viewed relations between parents and children primarily in terms of discipline and authority. This pre-war paradigm, grounded in behaviourism, stressed the importance of forming habits of behaviour necessary for productive life. During the Second World War anxiety about the impact on children of discipline and authority began to be expressed, the concern being that 'despotic' discipline could lead to the sort of nightmare society that Nazi Germany represented. Scholarly and professional discourses that spoke about the child as an individual, favoured a more democratic approach to child-rearing, and encouraged humane discipline of the child through guidance and understanding, helped popularise new ideals, eventually resulting in the birth of the 'permissive' culture (Jenkins, 1998). The 'permissive' model saw parent-child relations increasingly in terms of pleasure and play. Parents now had to relinquish traditional authority in order for children to develop autonomy and self-worth. In addition, whilst the pre-war model prepared children for the workplace within a society of scarcity, the post-war model prepared them to become pleasure-seeking consumers within a prosperous new economy (Wolfenstein, 1955).

Childhood, through a process of miniaturization, became a key metaphor through which adults spoke about their social and political concerns. Thus, permissiveness with regards child rearing allowed new identities to be prescribed not only for children, but also for adults. Mothers and fathers responded to this changing definition of childhood, seeing it as a vehicle for a fuller expression of themselves as parents. Parental obligations were reframed to pave the way for the culture of fun and permissiveness for all.

Following the traumas of the Second World War and the evacuation process for children in Britain, prominence was also given to the effects of early separation of young children from their mothers. This construction was reinforced by the development of attachment theory by the British psychoanalyst, John Bowlby. Separation, it was now claimed, produced an affectionless character that was the root cause of anti-social behaviour (Bowlby 1969, 1973).

Shifting economic structures were also leading to profound changes in the organization of family life. More mothers were employed outside the home, precipitating a renegotiation of power within the family. Suburbanization and the economic demands of successful market economies were resulting in greater mobility, less time for family life and a reduction of contact and exchanges between members of the extended family. Many families (particularly those headed by young women) were now isolated from traditional sources of childrearing information. Within this context childrearing guides took on an unprecedented importance, allowing for a more dramatic change in parenting styles than would have been conceivable in a more rooted community, and greater 'ownership' by professionals of the knowledge base for the task of parenting (Zuckerman, 1975).

The new child-centred permissive culture was a godsend to consumer capitalism, and gave rise to an industry of children's toys, books, and other 'educational' material (Weinman-Lear, 1963). The culture of consumption (with its expectations of a 'fun morality') became a major force shaping the child-rearing practices of the 20th century in the West. With the expansion of the consumer marketplace and suburban affluence, permissive conceptions of the child embraced pleasure as a positive motivation for exploration and learning.

Although a backlash against the culture of permissiveness took place, particularly in the 1980's and 90's, it was embedded in Western notions of childhood that put the individual at the centre and, following a period of decline in Western economies, was in service of capital. More parents were forced to work for longer hours, and state support, particularly for children and families, was harshly cut resulting in widespread child poverty and the creation of a new under-class.

With increasing numbers of households in which there were two working parents or single parents following divorce, fathers and mothers were less and less available for their children through the day. Left increasingly to their own devices children were more available to exploitation by the free market, which preyed on their boredom and desire for stimulation (Kincheloe, 1998). In such an environment, a media that tells them that they are deficient without this or that accessory constantly confronts children. Western children respond to these influences by entering early, and without adult supervision, into the world of adult entertainments, becoming sexually knowledgeable and with earlier experience of drugs and alcohol (Aronowitz and Giroux, 1991). This push by the market to 'adultify' them is matched by the effect of the culture of self-gratification that makes 'children' of adults. Many argue that, as a result, childhood in the West is being eroded, lost or indeed has suffering a strange death (Jenhs, 1996). It is claimed that childhood is disappearing as children have gained access to the world of adult information, resulting in a blurring of boundaries between adulthood and childhood, and leading in effect to children coming to be viewed as miniature adults. In such a context the idea of 'childhood innocence' comes to be viewed nostalgically, as something belonging to the past. Politicians have used this idea for their own purposes – for example, to extol the promise of a return to 'traditional family values' (Jenkins, 1998).

One result of these competing discourses and changes in family and lifestyle has been the development of some core tensions and ambivalence with regard children. The children's rights movements see 'childhood' as being at risk and needing strengthening by developing children's character and ability to reason, and safeguarding against pollution by adults. These activists often fail to notice how much the discourse of children's rights itself has eroded boundaries between adults and children. Processes that make children older than their years often accompany cries for childhood to be preserved. This contradiction runs through modern conceptions of childhood innocence; we both desire it and want to help children to move beyond it, we want to 'coddle' the child and we want to 'discipline' the child (Aries, 1998).

At the same time there has been a growing concern that children themselves have become the danger. They are viewed as deviant and violent troublemakers despite being the very generation who were given the best of everything (Seabrook, 1982; Alcock and Harris, 1982). At the end of the twentieth century our vision of childhood in the West was a polarized one, at one pole we have the victimized 'innocent' child who needs rescuing, and at the other pole we have the impulsive, aggressive, sexual child who is a threat to society. Equally polarized, parents are set impossible standards by those who set themselves up as protectors of children, and many are marginalized by child welfare professionals as potentially neglectful or abusive parents (Scheper-Hughes and Stein, 1987). Being viewed as a 'normal' child, or a 'normal' parent, have arguably, become, harder than ever to achieve.

The common thread through both these visions of 'childhood at risk', and of 'children as the risk', is the suggestion that modern society has seen a collapse of adult authority (morally and physically). This collapse is reflected in the growth in parental spending on children and the endless search by parents for emotional gratification for their children (Cunningham, 1995; Zelizer,

1985). As increasing concerns are voiced about children's development, so fingers have been pointed towards the role of the family, particularly mothers, towards the genetic make-up of the child, and the nature of schooling environments. Judgements about abnormal childhoods and family forms have become harsher and parents and children feel ever more closely scrutinized (Boyden, 1997; Winn, 1984; Morgan, 1987; Barlow and Hill, 1985). One result has been the mushrooming of explanations that locate the cause of the anxiety within the individual child, resulting in the development of a new reconstruction of childhood in primarily biological/genetic terms.

In chapter 3, Begum Maitra points out that Western notions of 'child-centredness' that dominate law and policy are no more 'progressive' or 'natural', nor are these 'superior' to the goals that non-Western cultures have devised with regard to their children. Imbued with the authority of 'expert' knowledge and applied without regard to the cultural and family context of the child, Western concepts are as likely to cause harm as do good. In her critique of so-called 'child-centred' practice Begum Maitra outlines processes in the West that have taken the bearing and rearing of children out of the 'natural' realm and into the professional realm of 'parenting' expertise, while heightening the apparent conflict between individual choice and 'traditional' notions – of parenthood, obligation and agency. The growing focus on children's rights, combined with parental anxiety that *any* influence that is *discernible* may be likely to be viewed as *undue* influence, makes it more likely that parents will leave essential socialising guidance to the expertise of professionals. She warns that an over-reliance on professional relationships for the ordinary losses, hurts and grievances that life necessarily brings may hinder our ability to develop the skills, and the sort of society, that support survival through these.

In chapter 7 Sami Timimi and Elisse Moody discuss how our under-standing of the 'institutional' child has changed. The chapter tries to track some of the key factors influencing Western societies changing visions and practices in relation to children deemed unfit or unable to continue living with their families because of deviance from the cultural norms of the time, in their behaviour, thoughts and/or feelings. Concentrating on the historical context that led, first to the birth, and then to the growth of psychiatric in-patient institutions for children and adolescents, they show how the nature of residential adolescent in-patient units can be understood as being a product of the social/political/economic/cultural conditions of the time. Just as each development can be situated within in its own historical context so the current situation with regard psychiatric in-patient institutions for children and adolescents does not represent some sort of end-point and is likely to change further as a result of social dynamics – such as changing economic, political and medical opinion.

In chapter 8 Eia Asen provides an account of past and current systemic practice. Different schools of thought and styles of practice have evolved slowly and steadily over the years, reflecting changing societal, cultural and political landscapes. He believes that as systemic practice nears a more mature age, multi-modal collaboration and attempted integration of different systemic approaches and techniques are becoming more common.

Non-Western childhoods

As well as changing visions of normal and deviant childhoods within cultures (vertically evidence), differences may be identified horizontally, that is, between different cultures at the same point in time. Broadly speaking the predominant differences between non-Western and Western approaches to children is visible in the prolonged indulgence accorded to infants, and in the earlier acceptance of certain adult responsibilities in many non-Western cultures. Thus, in Western cultures the search for evidence of independence, self-reliance and self-control starts more or less as soon as the child is born, while many non-Western cultures promote emotional dependence through immediate gratification of the child's perceived needs. As the child grows older in Western culture independence is encouraged in thinking style, verbal communication and emotional expression. Physical labour and the acceptance of duties and responsibilities do not occur until much later in Western as opposed to many non-Western cultures, to the extent that a new phase in child development emerged in the West, a phase between childhood and adulthood that we call adolescence. In many non-Western cultures adolescence as a clear life stage with its own sub-culture is not so readily apparent, while a movement into adult duties and responsibilities (that include the products of a child's physical labour, as well as an early introduction to spiritual duties) may be already apparent before the onset of puberty (Timimi, 2005).

In chapter 3, Begum Maitra examines the cultural smorgasbord that contemporary Western societies appear to offer. Within the relative affluence of the West, dominant discourses about choice confound attempts to elucidate the complex nature of cultural difference (both intra- and inter-cultural), and appear to suppress an ('ordinary', even matter of fact) awareness of disparity – whether economic, social, or of individual capacity. She points to the influences in non-Western cultures that have produced vastly different notions of children and their needs, and asks whether Western psychological theory makes any attempt to accommodate this diversity. Pointing to the rigidity of professional belief systems that are based at least in part on an outdated imperialism, Begum Maitra suggests that the cost to minority ethnic children and their families of continuing cultural incompetence among professionals is both significant and distressing.

In chapter 4 Rajeev Banhatti, Kedar Dwivedi and Begum Maitra explore the ways in which ideas about children developed in and around India. They point out that any attempt to encompass the history, politics, and religion, not to mention psychology, of a region so large and varied in a single chapter is always going to be only partially successful. Noting these limitations the authors pick out a small number of themes relevant to children, and illustrate how these may be traced back to the shared past of the people in the Indian subcontinent. From this past arose ideas about what made a good life, exemplary tales of children and their relationships, mythologies, and religious traditions that, filtered through memory and re-constructions, create the particular repertoire of contemporary beliefs and practices that make for an 'Indian' childhood. Cultural practices, even those most recently invented or borrowed, rarely have short histories. Although the chapter focuses on only one among the many South Asian cultures, and from among the numerous other world cultures that may be relevant to British clinicians, it does so without apology. The authors note that few papers that deal with clinical issues simultaneously address background cultural matters at any length. Lists of ethnic groups, languages, religious and dietary customs are of little help in understanding the detail of emotional lives and relationships. In their chapter, the authors have focused mainly on the traditional Hindu perspective. They explain that the ultimate goal of life, in this view, has for millennia been that of spiritual (rather than individual or material) development with the liberation of the soul from the cycle of birth and rebirth. An unbroken tradition of Indian thought describes children as complex entities from birth, and childhood as a gift of the divine life force. The ideologies behind parenting practices reflect these beliefs and goals, aiming to help the child transcend egotistic narcissism and toward the cultivation of dependability and interdependence (rather than towards independence). Mythology, as in tales of the childhood exploits of gods and heroes, provides both sources of shared entertainment and powerful role models for Indian children.

In chapter 8 Eia Asen points out that adopting systemic perspectives means viewing the child and his or her mental issues in a variety of contexts. These include not only the immediate and the wider family, but also the social and cultural setting of which the child and family are part. A systemic perspective also includes examining the relationship between the child, the family and the professional 'team' that constructs and/or diagnoses 'mental health issues' or psychiatric illness or disorder. Moreover, by working in multi-cultural settings, clinicians are learning that families from different ethnic and religious backgrounds require different interventions. He points out that, unfortunately, most systemic therapists working in public services adapt their approach to the work contexts and presenting problems, rather than the differing beliefs of the children and families they work with.

The more one learns how views of 'normal' childhood vary between different cultures, and within the same culture over time, the more difficult it becomes to assert a universal set of norms for childhood. Thus there can be no universal way of defining what behaviours should be considered as deviant. These are not differences of detail. From individual to family orientation, from prolonged indulgence to early independence, from the predominance of non-verbal to the dominance of the cognitive and verbal, from physical closeness to physical distance, from conformity to freedom of expression, from narrowly circumscribed expectations to a wider repertoire of accepted expressions, from spiritual centred-ness to scientific rationality, from ambivalence to conflict, from freedom of movement to close scrutiny, from gendered to non-gendered expectations, from duty and responsibility to play and stimulation – how would one decide which version is the normal? Which version is the universal healthy and natural childhood from which others have deviated?

The medicalisation of childhood

With the medical profession having played a central role in developing modern, Western ideas about child development and child rearing, it has been ideally placed both socially and politically, to respond to the current cultural anxiety about children and their childhoods. Using its status and position of power to further increase its own influence over children and families, paediatricians, child psychiatrists and psychologists, have chosen popular European post-enlightenment cultural preoccupations with reason and the individual subject, as well as being subject to the same market demands of increasing personal profitability. Thus context-deprived approaches that focus on the individual child, as the locus of this anxiety, with the idea that a chemical imbalance or neurological delay in development is the cause of a child's perceived problems, has become commonplace practice in the West. As with adult psychiatry no evidence of pathological lesions has been forth-coming and there are no psychological, neurological, or other physical markers to assist the clinician in making diagnoses of childhood and adolescent psychiatric disorder.

The need of market economies to expand continually has allowed drug companies to exploit these new, vague and broadly defined childhood psychiatric diagnoses, resulting in a rapid increase in the amount of psychotropic medication being prescribed to children and adolescents in the West. For example, the amount of psychotropic medication prescribed to children in the United States increased nearly four fold between 1985 and 1994 (Pincus et al, 1998). More recently researchers analyzing prescribing trends in nine countries (UK, France, Germany, Spain, Canada, USA, Argentina, Brazil, and Mexico), between 2000 and 2002, found significant rises in the number of prescriptions for psychotropic drugs in children, were evident in all countries-the lowest being in Germany where the increase was 13%, and the highest being in the UK where an increase of 68% was recorded (Wong et al, 2004).

Little research has been done on the safety and efficacy of psychotropic drugs in children, with prescribing patterns in children often being based on information drawn from research in adults (Wong et al, 2004). Of particular concern is the increase in rates of stimulant prescription to children. By 1996 over six percent of school-aged boys in the United States were taking stimulant medication (Olfson et al, 2002) with children as young as two being prescribed stimulants in increasing numbers (Zito et al, 2000). Recent surveys show that in some schools in the United States over seventeen percent of boys are taking stimulant medication (Le Fever et al, 1999). In the UK prescriptions for stimulants have increased from about 6,000 in 1994 to about 345,000 children in the latter half of 2003 (Wright, 2003), suggesting that we in the UK are rapidly catching up with the US.

With enormous profits to be made for the pharmaceutical industry, the combination of doctors carving out new roles for themselves together with aggressive marketing by the drug industry, a very powerful and difficult to resist combination has arisen. Privileged social groups, who hold important and influential positions, have a powerful effect on our common cultural beliefs, attitudes and practices. Child psychiatry in the UK does appear to have re-invented itself in the last 10 years. Powerful child psychiatrists successfully influenced the UK's professional discourse convincing it that there were more personal rewards for the profession by it adopting a more medicalised American style (e.g. Goodman, 1997). This has encouraged not only, the creation and widespread 'recognition' for new child psychiatric diagnoses, but also the construction of whole new classes of disorder- such as 'neurodevelopmental psychiatry', which the public, trusting such high status opinions, has come to view as real.

Modern child psychiatric practice in North America has been characterised as having symptom based, context deprived assessments, using multiple screening questionnaires, aggressive use of psychotropic medication and use of multiple prescriptions often with little information about safety or long-term consequences (Pincus et al, 1998). As with adult psychiatry this places child psychiatry in a symbiotic discourse with the political establishment. Not only do we continue to make fundamental contributions to everyday thinking about what is normal and abnormal for children and parenting, but we also volunteer ourselves as powerful agents of social control.

In Chapter 2 Jon Jureidini and Peter Mansfield discuss the role drug companies have had in the greater medicalisation of childhood problems that we have witnessed in recent decades in the West. Pharmaceutical companies use the most effective promotional methods that they can to increase sales income. They have an obligation to maximise profit for shareholders, as well as self-interest in maximising income for their company. Thus the hard sell is an inevitable consequence of the way that drug companies are paid and it would be too simplistic to blame drug companies for what is really a systems problem. However, they note that such promotion has an adverse effect on health outcomes. Pharmaceutical companies do not just promote drugs; they also promote illness (which, of course, leads to the increased sale of drugs). They do this by sponsoring or producing material for general practitioners, doctor's waiting rooms and others that alert the medical and lay community to the existence of 'new' conditions like 'social phobia', or 'under diagnosed' ones, like 'dysthymia', and investing in consumer support groups that promote similar messages.

Although it has never been recommended by the Royal Colleges in Britain and/or other authorities, that anti-depressants be used as first line treatment for childhood depression, both Sami Timimi (chapter 10) and Jon Jureidini and Peter Mansfield (chapter 2) claim that in practice they have already achieved that status. Jon Jureidini and Peter Mansfield (chapter 2) believe that a significant contribution to this level of prescribing is that general practitioners are the primary prescribers of anti-depressants. Writing a prescription is quick and easy. GPs rarely have the time and training to provide much non- drug therapy and often feel strongly the need to 'do something' quickly to reduce the risk of suicide, as well as reduce the suffering. Furthermore, GPs decision-making often depends heavily on clinical experience, and they may tend to attribute improvements to their prescriptions. Thus many GPs see anti-depressant prescribing as the best or the only treatment in their repertoire for childhood depression. Sami Timimi (chapter 10) argues that the gateway diagnosis to prescribing anti-depressants is that of 'childhood depression', a diagnosis that he believes helps medicalise childhood unhappiness and has the effect of cutting the child off from their context. A mutually beneficial relationship between certain academic psychiatrists and the drug industry has developed where the psychiatrists provide the drug companies with the tools and the drug company, by promoting their products, implicitly endorse the validity of the concepts for which their product is being marketed as a 'treatment'. A shift in theory and consequently practice then took place, as influential academics claimed that childhood depression was more common than previously thought, resembled adult depression, and was amenable to treatment with anti-depressants.

A critique of the evidence supporting a biomedical model

In chapter 6 Jonathan Leo refers to 'Confusion, manipulation, and institutional failure' which was the recent summary on *The Lancet's* editorial page about the research into selective serotonin reuptake inhibitor (SSRI) use in childhood depression (Editors, 2004). The editors' conclusions were based on revelations that pharmaceutical companies had selectively reported favourable research about the use of antidepressants in children. However, he also believes that the medical community makes a mistake if it believes that the current problem is just one of unpublished data, which the pharmaceutical companies have kept hidden. Jonathan Leo argues that the system of academic medicine failed. It failed to the point that the academic journals were circulating a myth about the benefits of psychotropic drugs that had little to do with the evidence. He then considers two cases where mainstream medicine and its institutions (such as medical schools, medical journals, and government research organizations) have failed to adequately confront and critically appraise prevailing accepted evidence that support the idea that distressed children need pharmacological interventions. One case involves the revelations about the discrepancies between unpublished and published data on antidepressant use in children. The second case relates to institutional biases when it comes to the interpretation of data generated from neuroimaging studies comparing medicated ADHD children to unmedicated ADHD children.

In chapter 10 Sami Timimi points out that from a purely scientific point of view, it is hard to understand how childhood depression as a diagnosis has come into existence and why it is diagnosed so frequently. He notes that co-morbidity in childhood depression is high, there are questions as to whom and on what basis one decides where the cut-off mark is between 'normal' and 'pathological' is, that having a categorical diagnosis bears only a tenuous relationship with level of psychosocial impairment, that childhood depression is only weakly associated with suicide, that 'biological markers' do not work with children and adolescents diagnosed as depressed, that separating environmental from biological factors in the familial clustering has been virtually impossible, that the postulated continuity of childhood depression with adulthood depression comes from studies with serious methodological flaws, and that children do not show many of the symptoms said to be common in adult depression and instead are said to show more non-specific symptoms such as irritability, running away from home, decline in schoolwork and headaches.

In chapter 9 Sami Timimi argues that economically and politically powerful groups (drug companies, doctors and teachers) have had a major, but often unacknowledged, impact on a local communities conception concerning the nature of childhood, resulting in a new category of childhood emerging- that of the ADHD child. He notes that the diagnosis of attention deficit hyperactivity disorder (ADHD) has reached epidemic proportions, particularly amongst boys in the West and documents an alarming rise in the amount of potentially addictive medications these children are receiving. He discusses the history behind the growth of the idea of a 'neurodevelopmental' disorder called ADHD suggesting that the popularisation of ADHD has more to do with our changing ideas about the nature of childhood than any scientific breakthrough. In this sense ADHD can be thought of as a cultural response to a culture specific perception of a social crisis with regard children and their behaviour. Reviewing the evidence in favour firstly of conceptualizing ADHD as a medical disorder and secondly of using stimulants to 'treat' this, he concludes on both counts that the evidence is unconvincing. Furthermore the widespread concerns about stimulants safety, which should be considered as important information for all parents trying to make the difficult decision as to whether or not to agree for their children to take a stimulant, is information that is rarely given by prescribers.

David Woodhouse notes in chapter 11 that for the past 40 years the majority of the medical establishment has ignored the possible link between nutrition and physical disease states. Similarly, the mental health community has followed their lead, with mainstream psychiatry and psychology maintaining there is little relationship between nutrition and mental health. Yet a review of the literature reveals that, for virtually every major mental condition, studies exists demonstrating that there are significant nutritional influences.

In chapter 5 Charles Whitfield points out that there is a large body of literature showing a link between childhood trauma or abuse and subsequent behaviour problems including ADHD-type behaviours, violence and aggression. He notes that many who are erroneously diagnosed with ADHD/ADD – and some who are accurately diagnosed with it – may have a history of abuse or trauma that has been overlooked. In his literature search he found 77 published reports of a significantly higher incidence of ADHD type behaviours and ADHD among abused children and found only one study that looked for it that reported a negative association of ADHD with trauma. He also found 66 studies that reported an association between violent and aggressive behaviour and having a history of childhood trauma/abuse. Charles Whitfield concludes that childhood trauma can lead to a multitude of health and social problems including those that result from disrupted development of the brain and nervous system as a result of the physical effects of chronic stress on the developing brain.

The implication for children and society

Without good evidence to support the idea that these new diagnoses are the result of physical pathology, the medicalisation of the West's views on child development and child rearing, is best understood as the West's most recent way of interpreting how children should be, rather than the result of scientific endeavour that is leading us ever closer to the 'truth' about the universal nature of childhood. Just as we may look back with a critical eye at previous generations' assumptions about the nature of child development, there is no reason to assume that we have reached some final end-point in our current assumptions, and that we will not similarly be criticised by future generations. To conclude that our current Western views of child development are socially constructed (in other words we are creating not discovering the meanings we give to children's behaviour and emotional state) is not enough; we still have to critique the utility to children, families, and society of the preferred meanings we give.

Within Western child developmental discourse there is a constant subtext that is saying there is a superior and inferior position. Development says to the child, the parent and the teacher this is your future and if you do not reach it you are, in some senses, inferior (Morss, 1996). It is not just children who are said to develop but also peoples and economies (Rahman, 1993; Sachs, 1992). Development is about modern hierarchies of superiority and inferiority – it is about dismissing diversity. Developmental explanations instil the notion of individual competitiveness; from the moment you are born you will have developmental milestones thrust upon you. As parents we are desperate to see our children achieve these age bound expectations. Development of our children is under constant professional surveillance starting with health visitors and community paediatricians and moving on to general practitioners, nursery nurses, teachers and the whole range of para-psycho-medicine specialists. We are concerned when our children seem to be falling behind and we are constantly encouraging them to achieve these expectations. If we are not concerned and not encouraging, presumably we are neglecting.

How does this affect the children themselves? If there is a belief that these are natural, unfolding processes for which professionals must be involved in helping children achieve, does this not encourage competitiveness from a very early age? How much do children get caught in these parental and professional anxieties? How relaxed can children, from the moment they are born be to just be, as opposed to having to do something to ease these cultural anxieties? When these anxieties cannot be comforted and there is a perception that a child has strayed from their pre-destined developmental path, which is to blame? In this blame ridden culture that needs an explanation for everything much of the developmental psychopathology literature has generally pointed toward the mother for blame and more recently toward the child's genes. In a culture where families have shrunk and fathers seem to disappear and relinquish duty and responsibility in ever increasing numbers, mothers often have to shoulder not only the responsibility for caring for their family (a role given much lower status in Western culture than many non-Western cultures), but also for things going wrong. In a final stab from the developmental discourse mothers are then denied credit for their work when things do go well as children are then simply seen as achieving their biological destiny.

Within this context the more bio-deterministic aspects of the developmental and developmental psychopathology culture has, at least, appeared to provide a get-out clause for the beleaguered mother. Now problems can be viewed as being the result of a fault in the genetic programme for development and thus intrinsic to the child. But this approach to understanding the problems of children is equally guilty in its simplistic theoretical assumptions, and in denying alternative possibilities. Furthermore, it never solves the nagging doubt in the back of a parent's mind that it is their fault, leads to children internalising a potentially lifelong personal script of disability (with its potential for disconnecting a person from their own capacity for agency), and exposes children to a plethora of untested, possibly harmful, psychotropic medications.

Western child development/psychiatric disorder beliefs heavily influence the education system our children grow up in. For example the defining of a disability requiring special needs help at school is shaped by the disciplines of medicine and psychology (Hey, et al, 1998). The adherence of these two fields to measuring physical and mental competence in order to determine normality inevitably conveys assumptions about deviance and failure and these labels then become attached to both individuals and groups which have failed to measure up/conform. Special needs practice within schools rests on within child explanations (Ainscow and Tweddle, 1988) and on the whole are focused upon reading ability or acting out behaviour (Daniels, et al, 1998). There are important gender differences with special needs resources in schools going to a much higher proportion of boys than girls (Daniels, et al, 1998). There are also obvious differences in special needs provision within schools by race, with black pupils appearing to be systematically diverted from the category of specific reading difficulties and allocated to mild to moderate learning difficulties and black boys in particular to emotional and behavioural difficulties, while white boys tend to dominate the reading support resources (Hey, et al, 1998). Like the professions of psychology and psychiatry, teaching has fallen victim of rationalist, scientific, market values and has moved toward a more 'technicist' approach, with greater emphasis on specialisation and less acknowledgement of the human social exchange nature of a teacher's activity, leading to: deskilling and greater emotional detachment from their work (Skelton, 2001), the return of more didactic beliefs and practices in school that revolve around concepts derived from a child development perspective, and an increase in the number of children referred by schools for medical management (usually with medication) of behaviour problems (Timimi, 2005).

Then there is the problem of colonialism. Western attitudes and beliefs with regard child rearing are being exported to countries conceptualized as 'underdeveloped' (in moral/ethical/knowledge as well as economic spheres) and taken up by local professionals many of whom understandably believe they are getting something better from the more sophisticated and advanced West. For example the *Handbook of Asian Child Development and Child Rearing Practices* (Suvannathat, 1985), prepared by Thia child development experts, is highly influenced by Western medico-psychological ideology. The book sets out to assimilate Western child development theory into a third world context with very little evidence of taking a local perspective into account. Thus the authors suggest that many of the traditional beliefs and practices of

Asians prevent them from seeking and using new scientific knowledge in child rearing, and go on to argue, in line with Western thinking, that children should be given more independence with less use of power and authority by the parents.

Just as problematic notions of child rearing are being imposed on countries of the South, so also are problematic notions of child mental health problems. Economically and politically powerful groups, such as the doctors and the pharmaceutical industry, have enabled Western medicine to push back its frontiers of influence. Rapid growth in the prescribing of psychotropic medications to children is happening in many countries of the South (such as Brazil and Mexico) (Wong et al, 2004), suggesting the Western individualized biological/genetic conception of childhood mental health problems is spreading to the countries of the South and may be undermining more helpful indigenous belief systems with regard the problems of childhood (Timimi, 2002, 2005).

Begum Maitra (chapter 3) believes that the costs to minority ethnic children, and their families, of continuing cultural incompetence among professionals is distressingly large, pointing out that the rigidity of existing professional belief systems are based, at least in part, on an outdated imperialism, and on an insistence on using Western paradigms of what it is to be 'human'. She also cautions about the temptation to make unjustifiable claims for the mental health disciplines inspired by a political climate of endless 'innovation', and to periodically weigh up the validity and impact of our intrusions into private relationships. She quotes Archard (1993: 120) warning against an overemphasis on the privacy of the family, "*Against that, arguments to the effect that the public can be familialised, that is that all our social relationships can be transformed to resemble a large family are simply naïve*", and wonders if this seems a better solution than an over-reliance on professional relationships for the ordinary losses, hurts and grievances that life necessarily brings.

In chapter 4 Rajeev Banhatti, Kedar Dwivedi and Begum Maitra discuss that in the context of British colonialism in India, progress was conceptualised as a reformation of the *childlike* Indian (innocent, ignorant but willing to learn, loyal and grateful) by 'Westernisation', modernisation or Christianisation or of the *childish* Indian (ignorant but unwilling to learn, ungrateful, sinful, savage, disloyal and incorrigible) by repression, brutal force and tough rule of law and administration. One can of course see echoes or continuity of this imperialistic thinking in international politics even today. The colonisation of Indian minds was probably more damaging in the long term and in many ways Indians had to search for the unique Indian self in themselves even after the outward war of Independence was won in 1947. The pressure to be the obverse of the West distorts the traditional priorities in the Indians' views of themselves; it in fact binds them even more irrevocably to the West. On the other hand, child rearing practices and the childcare techniques have been practised over Indian subcontinents for thousands of years from generations to generations with minor changes in different regions and culture. However, no notable bad effects are observed. This has more importance in the light of behavioural disturbances found in children from the West. Although this needs to be seen in the context of other socioeconomic realities (such as, high infant mortality) and reports of female infanticide, it makes one wonder whether some aspects of Indian culture somehow lead to greater resilience in children. If this is so, they ask, how is it transmitted to the children and how might we in the West learn something positive for both our conceptions of healthy child rearing and treatment in Western child and adolescent mental health services?

Eia Asen (chapter8) suggests that Child and Adolescent Mental Services have well-established institutional practices. Children, teenagers and their families tend to get fairly similar assessments and treatments, no matter what their presentations, their problem history or their ethnicity. What is 'on offer' is said to be determined by the children's and families' perceived or postulated 'needs', as well as by the respective trainings and skills of the staff. The term 'need', so frequently used, requires some discussion. Who actually defines 'need'? Do professionals identify certain 'needs' so that their interventions 'fit'? He points out that 'need' is a social construction; it is not 'real' as such.

Jon Jureidini and Peter Mansfield (chapter 2) point out that the negative effects on health from the promotion of new drugs include; direct harm from inferior efficacy, increased adverse effects (some only emerge after years on the market), inappropriate use because of unfamiliarity, and the rising cost of drugs, diverting funds from other high priority areas at a time when health sector funding is reaching crisis point.

Sami Timimi (chapters 9 and 10) suggests that there may be a real increase in unhappiness being experienced by children having to grow up in a Western cultural context that has seen huge changes in child rearing practices, family structure, lifestyle, and education. Context-deprived paradigms such as child-hood depression and ADHD that conceptualise problems in individualistic terms and therefore lead to individualistic interventions (such as pharmacotherapy and cognitive therapy), render more context-rich interventions such as family and systemic therapies to the margins. What a context-deprived approach allows our profession to collude with, are the de-politicisation of children's difficulties and the obscuring of the changing challenges facing children and their families in modern Western capitalist societies. Thus the real life circumstances that children and young people face need integrating into a multi-perspective approach that engages with the interpersonal realities experienced and the new possible meanings that can be generated when the reliance on reductionist models that emphasise pathology are abandoned in favour of more positive and multi-dimensional approaches.

In chapter 11 David Woodhouse describes the work of the Cactus Clinic, which provides a novel non-drug treatment approach for children diagnosed with ADHD. He points out that many parents who came to the clinic had been told that, unless they placed their child on medication, there was nothing else that the medical profession could do for them as this was the only treatment on offer for ADHD. Other parents had been told that if they wanted their child to remain in school then they must put him/her on a medication programme, and those who had followed the medical advice were given little or no information about the potential side effects of that medication. Similarly, parents with children on the medication programme had seen these side effects and wanted to take their child off medication.

In chapter 5 Charles Whitfield argues that abused and neglected children are hurt by trauma, and yet are often misdiagnosed by ascribing their difficulties to something intrinsic to them (such as ADHD). Rather than address these effects appropriately as being caused by the trauma, many authority figures such as parents, teachers, law enforcement people, and doctors may unwittingly label and therefore blame the child, which in effect re-victimizes them further and decreases their already low self-esteem. How helpful, he asks, is it to label children with disorders such as 'ADHD' when, instead, the child's behaviour may be a normal reaction to a difficult/stressful environment that they find themselves in.

SUMMARY

In this book we have gathered together a number of authors who, like us, wish to critique some of the fundamental assumptions upon which current theory and practice in child and adolescent mental health is based. The chapters present the ideas of different authors that explore the social construction of childhood distress, some of the cultural and political dynamics behind common child psychiatric assumptions, evaluate the evidence for the current popular concepts used in child and adolescent psychiatry, discuss the implications for children and society of the uncritical acceptance of current theory and practice, and provide ideas on alternative ways of working. The challenge now is how to bring some of these debates into the mainstream where they undoubtedly belong.

References

Ainscow, M. and Tweddle, D.A. (1988) *Encouraging Classroom Success*. London: Fulton.

Alcock, P. and Harris, P. (1982) *Welfare, Law and Order: A Critical Introduction to Law for Social Workers*. London: MacMillan.

Archard, D. (1993) *Children Rights and Childhood*. London: Routledge.

Aries, P. (1998) From immodesty to innocence. In H Jenkins (ed.) *Children's Culture Reader*. New York: New York University Press.

Aronowitz, S. and Giroux, H. (1991) *Post-modern Education: Politics, Culture and Social Criticism*. Minneapolis: University of Minnesota Press.

Barlow, G. and Hill, A. (1985) *Video Violence and Children*. London: Hodder and Stoughton.

Bowlby, J. (1969) *Attachment and Loss, Volume 1, Attachment*. London: Hogarth Press.

Bowlby, J. (1973) *Attachment and Loss, Volume 2, Separation*. London: Hogarth Press.

Boyden, J. (1997) 'Childhood and the policy makers: A comparative perspective on the globalization of childhood' in A. James and A. Prout (eds.) *Constructing and Reconstructing Childhood*. London: Falmer Press.

Bracken, P. and Thomas, P. (2001) Post psychiatry: a new direction for mental health. *British Medical Journal* 322, 724-727.

Calvert, K. (1992) *Children in the House: The Material Culture of Early Childhood, 1600-1900*. Boston: Northeastern University Press.

Clarke, J., Hall, S., Jefferson, T. and Roberts, B. (1975) 'Subcultures, culture and subcultures' in S. Hall and T. Jefferson (eds.) *Resistance Through Rituals: Youth Subcultures in Post-War Britain*. London: Hutchinson.

Coles, R. (1986) *The Political Life of Children*. Boston: Atlantic monthly press.

Cunningham, H. (1995) *Children and Childhood in Western Society Since 1500*. London: Longman.

Daniels, H., Hey, V., Leonard, D. and Smith, M. (1998) Difference, difficulty and equity: Gender race and SEN. *Management in Education* 12, 5-8.

Durkheim, E. (1925) *Moral Education: A Study in the Theory and Application of the Sociology of Education*. Translated by E.K. Wilson and H. Schnurer. New York: Free Press of Glancoe (1961).

Editors (2004) Depressing research. *The Lancet* 363, 1335

Goodman, R. (1997) An over extended remit. *British Medical Journal* 314, 813-814.

Harkness, S. and Super, C. (Eds) (1996) *Parents' Cultural Belief Systems: Their origins, expressions and consequences*. London: Guilford Press.

Hendrick, H. (1997) 'Constructions and reconstructions of British childhood: An interpretive survey, 1800 to the present' in A. James and A. Prout (eds.) *Constructing and Reconstructing Childhood: Contemporary Issues in the Sociological Study of Childhood*. London: Falmer Press.

Hey, V., Leonard, D., Daniels, H. and Smith, M. (1998) 'Boys' underachievement, special needs practices and questions of equity' in D. Epstein, J. Elwood, V. Hey and J. Maw (eds.) *Failing Boys? Issues in Gender and Underachievement.* Buckingham: Open University Press.

Jenhs, C. (1996) *Childhood.* London: Routledge.

Jenkins, H. (1998) 'Introduction: Childhood Innocence and Other Modern Myths' in H. Jenkins (ed.) *The Children's Culture Reader.* New York: New York University Press.

Kincheloe, J. (1998) 'The new childhood; Home alone as a way of life' in H. Jenkins (ed.) *Children's Culture Reader.* New York: New York University Press.

LeFever, G.B., Dawson, K.V., & Morrow, A.D. (1999) The extent of drug therapy for attention deficit hyperactivity disorder among children in public schools. *American Journal of Public Health* 89, 1359-1364.

Morgan, P. (1987) *Delinquent Fantasies.* London: Temple Smith.

Morss, J.R. (1996) *Growing Critical: Alternatives To Developmental Psychology.* London & New York: Routledge.

Olfson, M., Marcus, S.C., Weissman, M.M. and Jensen, P.S. (2002) National trends in the use of psychotropic medications by children. *Journal of the American Academy of Child and Adolescent Psychiatry* 41, 514-21.

Pincus, H.A., Tanielian, T.L. and Marcus, S.C. (1998) Prescribing trends in psychotropic medications. *Journal of the American Medical Association* 279, 526-531.

Prout, A. and James, A. (1997) 'A new Paradigm for the sociology of childhood? Provenance, promise and problems' in A. James and A. Prout (eds.) *Constructing And Re-Constructing Childhood: Contemporary Issues In The Sociological Study Of Childhood.* London: Falmer Press.

Rahman, A. (1993) *People's Self-Development.* London: Zed Press.

Sachs, W. (1992) *The Developmental Dictionary.* London: Zed Press.

Scheper-Hughes, N. and Stein, H.F. (1987) 'Child abuse and the unconscious in American popular culture' in N. Scheper-Hughes (ed.) *Child Survival.* New York: D. Reidel Publishing.

Seabrook, J. (1982) *Working Class Childhood: An Oral History.* London: Gollancz.

Skelton, C. (2001) *Schooling the Boys: Masculinities and Primary Education.* Buckingham: Open University Press.

Suvannathat, C., Bhanthumnavin, D., Bhuapirom, L. and Keats, D.M. (eds.) (1985) *Handbook Of Asian Child Development And Child Rearing Practices.* Bangkok: Srina Kharinwirot University, Behavioural Science Research Institute.

Timimi, S. (2002) *Pathological Child Psychiatry And The Medicalization Of Childhood.* London: Brunner. Routledge.

Timimi, S. (2004) Rethinking childhood depression. *British Medical Journal* 329, 1394-1396.

Timimi, S. (2005) *Naughty Boys: Anti-social behaviour, ADHD and the role of culture.* Basingstoke: Palgrave MacMillan.

Timimi, S. and Taylor, E. (2004) ADHD is best understood as a cultural construct. *British Journal of Psychiatry* 184, 8-9.

Winn, M. (1984) *Children Without Childhood.* Harmondsworth: Penguin.

Wolfenstein, M. (1955) 'Fun morality: An analysis of recent child-training literature' in M. Mead and M. Wolfenstein (eds.) *Childhood in Contemporary Cultures.* Chicago: The University of Chicago Press.

Wong, I.C., Murray, M.L., Camilleri-Novak, D. & Stephens, P. (2004) Increased prescribing trends of paediatric psychotropic medications. *Archives of Disease in Childhood* 89, 1131-1132.

Wright, O. (2003) Ritalin use and abuse fears. *The Times (UK)* July 28th, 3.

Zelizer, V.A. (1985) *Pricing The Priceless Child: The Changing Social Value Of Children.* New York: Basic Books Inc.

Zito, J.M., Safer, D.J., Dosreis, S., Gardner, J.F., Boles, J. and Lynch, F. (2000) Trends in prescribing of psychotropic medication in pre-schoolers. *Journal of the American Medical Association* 283, 1025-30.

Zuckerman, M. (1975) Dr. Spock: The Confidence Man. In S. Kaplan & C. Rosenberg (eds.) *The Family in History.* Philadelphia: University of Pennsylvania Press.

2

The scope of the problem of the relationship between drug companies and doctors

Jon Jureidini · Peter Mansfield

Drug Promotion

It is clear that drugs are not always used in a way that optimises health. The contribution to this problem from pharmaceutical promotion is exemplified by the decision-making shortcut 'newer is better'. Newer drugs are more profitable for drug companies but more expensive for taxpayers and patients because of patent monopoly protection. Using the 'newer is better' short cut works well for choosing many consumer goods, such as vegetables and computers. However that shortcut often misleads when choosing drugs because the majority of new drugs are less cost effective than older ones. The percentage of new drugs that have any advantage over older cheaper drugs has been assessed as only 23% during 1989-2000 in the USA and only 10.5% during 1980-2003 in France (National Institute for Health Care Management, 2002; Industrial interests versus public health: the gap is growing- report, 2004).

The negative effects on health from the promotion of new drugs include:-

1 Direct harm from inferior efficacy, increased adverse effects (some only emerge after years on the market) or inappropriate use because of unfamiliarity.

2 The rising cost of drugs that diverts funds from other high priority areas at a time when health sector funding is reaching crisis point.

Pharmaceutical companies use the most effective promotional methods that they can to increase sales income. They have an obligation to maximise profit for shareholders, as well as self-interest in maximising income for staff and for the company as a whole (Estes, 1996). If companies do not perform competitively, and grow, they get taken over. These forces acting on drug companies mean that priority is often given to short-term performance at the expense of longer term considerations. Drug companies have little choice but to do whatever works to increase the sales of more expensive drugs, regardless of the impact on health care. Thus the hard sell is an inevitable consequence of the way that drug companies are paid. It is incorrect to blame drug companies for what is really a system problem (Jureidini and Mansfield, 2001).

Unfortunately such promotion has an adverse effect on health outcomes. A study of 109 advertisements in 10 leading medical journals found that 44% would lead to improper treatment if relied upon (Wilkes et al, 1992). Many doctors say that they are not influenced by such promotion. However, those of us who feel immune from this misinformation may be especially vulnerable (Sagarin et al, 2002). Orlowski and Wateska studied hospital doctors who denied that going to all expenses paid seminars at popular vacation sites would influence them. However, these doctors who claimed to be immune from such influence did significantly increase their prescribing of the promoted drugs starting from immediately after they received their invitations (Orlowski and Wateska, 1992). In another study, Stelfox et al showed that authors supporting the use of calcium channel antagonists were significantly more likely to have a financial relationship with manufacturers of these drugs (Stelfox et al, 1998).

Disease Promotion

Pharmaceutical companies do not just promote drugs, they also promote illness (which of course leads to increased sale of drugs) (Moynihan, 1998). They do this by sponsoring or producing material for GPs, doctor's waiting rooms and others that alert the medical and lay community to the existence of 'new' conditions like social phobia, or 'under-diagnosed' ones, like dysthymia. Moncrieff described a systematic Public Relations (PR) operation promoting social anxiety disorder as a disease. The campaign was targeted both directly to the community and to the psychiatric profession (Moncrieff, 2004). A favoured means of promoting new illnesses is for drug companies to invest in consumer support groups. Medawar and Hardon claim that the National Alliance for the mentally ill received over 11 million U.S. dollars from 18 pharmaceutical companies between 1996 and mid 1999 (Medawar and Hardon, 2004). It is cost effective for drug companies to invest in such groups without any direct promotion of their product (or indeed of drug therapy). The support groups increase the number of patients who present to doctors with ready made diagnoses. One advantage for pharmaceutical companies in using these forms of promotion is that they do not need to make a direct connection between the illness and their product. This allows them to present what they are doing as community service. The reason that they do not need to link their products to this covert promotional material is that their detailers' orthodox promotional programmes, apparently independently, but often in a well organised way, have already 'educated' us doctors, so that we are ready and willing to prescribe for these disorders. Of course we doctors may collude with this process, by being too ready to redefine patients' dissatisfaction with their predicaments and/or unsatisfactory lives as depression. Giving patients antidepressants can be a way for us to avoid confronting their misery.

There is also considerable opportunity for hidden promotion in the funding of research. For example, many so-called research studies are primarily designed to familiarise doctors with drugs and encourage their use, rather than to contribute to scientific knowledge. This may be particularly the case where doctors are flattered (and financially rewarded) by invitations to participate in international, multi-centred trials. Invited centres are not always required to make any real scientific contribution to the process. Readers might have had similar experiences to the first author who has been approached to participate in multi-centre trials of an SSRI. On one occasion he was asked to be 'chief investigator' for a trial of a drug for Obsessive Compulsive Disorder. He was offered this status if he could provide patients, even though he had no particular expertise in the area being researched, or in conducting drug trials.

Case Study: anti-depressants in children.

Recent studies suggest that the evidence of benefit from the use of anti-depressants in children is very thin. As we have described elsewhere, for a total of 477 patients treated in six studies (≥23% dropouts), of 42 reported measures, only 14 showed a statistical advantage for an antidepressant (Jureidini et al, 2004a). None of the 10 measures relying on patient- or parent-reported outcomes showed significant advantage for an antidepressant, so that claims for effectiveness were based entirely on ratings by doctors. No data regarding rates of self-harm attempts, presentations to emergency or mental health services, or school attendance were presented in any study. We concluded that investigators have exaggerated the benefits and downplayed the adverse effects of newer antidepressants in childhood depression. Improvement in control groups was strong so that additional benefit from drugs was of doubtful clinical significance. A Lancet systematic review published the next week supported our conclusions by finding that unpublished trials showed that newer antidepressants were even less effective and more harmful for children than suggested by the published trials (Craig et al, 2004). Later in 2004, the Treatment of Adolescent Depression Study (TADS) was used to promote use of fluoxetine for depressed children. TADS was funded by a US government agency but was conducted by investigators who have received industry funding. The investigators claimed to show an advantage for fluoxetine, especially when combined with Cognitive-Behaviour Therapy (TADS Team, 2004). However there were flaws in the way they reported their data (Jureidini et al, 2004b). TADS includes: a double-blind comparison of fluoxetine (109 subjects) vs. placebo (112); and an unblinded comparison between CBT alone (111) and fluoxetine+ CBT (107). The lack of patient-blinding and placebo-control in the latter two groups is likely to exaggerate the benefit seen in the fluoxetine + CBT group, who receive more face-to-face contact and knew (as did their doctors) that they were not receiving placebo. Comparing results across all four groups is therefore misleading. The authors' claim that a CBT + placebo arm would have been 'both too expensive and too artificial to have clinical relevance' is unconvincing. Invalid comparisons are neither value for money nor relevant. The valid finding from TADS is the lack of a statistical advantage of fluoxetine over placebo on the primary endpoint, the Children's Depression Rating Scale (CDRS-R; $p = 0.10$) but this was not mentioned in the abstract. Despite small numbers and the exclusion of known suicidal behaviour, TADS found a trend to more suicidal behaviour (6 attempts in the fluoxetine groups, versus 1 in the no-fluoxetine groups), consistent with other trials of SSRIs. Putting together that result with the lack of clinically significant advantage to drug over placebo on most measures, the benefits of fluoxetine, like all other antidepressants, are of doubtful clinical importance for children.

Professor Jane Garland, a participant in the Sertraline trials who became sceptical about their methodology and reporting, writes "The high placebo response of SSRIs may reinforce physician prescribing, and it has been difficult for many physicians to accept that SSRIs may be ineffective. A complicating factor is that the public at large has now accepted the model of depression as a chemical imbalance for which medication is the treatment of choice, and the physician may experience pressure to prescribe. The disappointing reality is that antidepressant medications have minimal to no effectiveness in childhood depression beyond a placebo effect". (Garland, 2004: 490) Compare, for example, the management of hypertension. A major trial in this area showed the average systolic blood pressure dropped from 170 mm Hg to 155 mm Hg for the placebo group and 143 mm Hg for the active treatment group; average diastolic blood pressure from 77 mm Hg to 72 and 68 mm Hg, respectively (SHEP Cooperative Research Group, 1991). That is, blood pressure was down 15/5 with placebo and down 27/9 in the low dose chlorthalidone group, so that 55% of the effect of seen in the group taking the drug is also seen in the group taking the placebo. The difference between the average end point in the treatment group and the average end point in the placebo group is clinically significant. For comparison, Wagner and colleagues in a study of childhood depression with Sertraline found an average decrease on the Children's Depression Rating Scale-Revised of 23 points with Sertraline and 20 points with placebo (Wagner et al, 2003). Thus for depression, 85% of the improvement seen in the drug group was also seen in the placebo group. Furthermore the 3 point advantage for the drug group over that reached by the placebo group on a scale which has a range of 17 to 113 is of dubious clinical advantage.

It has never been recommended by colleges and other authorities that anti-depressants be first line treatment for childhood depression, yet in practice they have already achieved that status. A large American data set showed the prevalence of antidepressant use among children to have increased from 1.6% in 1998 to 2.4% in 2002, an annual increase of over 9%. In the 15 – 18 year old female age group the prevalence of antidepressant use was 6.4% (Delate et al, 2002). A significant contribution to this level of prescribing is that General Practitioners are the primary prescribers of anti-depressants. Children with depression are more likely to be seen by GPs than child psychiatrists. There are long delays for appointments with child psychiatrists. Psychologists are expensive because they are not subsidised and there has been little promotion of psychologists as suitable referral destinations for children with depression. Yet Hollinghurst et al (2005) have shown in adults that the money spent on higher levels of antidepressant prescribing in the NHS in 2002 compared with 1991 could have been used to deliver psychological services to more than a third of patients with depression. But writing a prescription is quick and easy. GPs rarely have the time and training to provide much non- drug therapy. Importantly, GPs feel strongly the need to 'do something' quickly to reduce the risk of suicide, as well as reduce the suffering. GPs decision making often depends heavily on clinical experience and we tend to attribute improvements to our prescriptions. Thus many GPs see anti-depressant prescribing as the best or the only treatment in their repertoire for childhood depression. There is also sometimes strong pressure from parents on GPs to prescribe.

Misleading presentation of research data

Advocates for the use of antidepressants claim support from research. But the available research has been shown to be questionable on the following grounds:-

1. Limited availability of research findings. Unpublished data gives a more pessimistic view of the effectiveness of anti-depressants in children (Craig et al, 2004). In 1998, the management of GlaxoSmithKline instructed staff to withhold clinical trial findings indicating that Paroxetine had no beneficial effect for adolescents with depression (Kondro and Sibbald, 2004). As Zito et al point out; no clinical trial is finished until the data are made available (Zito et al, 2004). They note that the sponsors and investigators bear risk but it is 'the subjects who bear the greatest risks; thus, they should also receive the benefits' (Zito et al, 2004: 513). Zito et al go on to advocate a registry of all paediatric psychopharmacology trials be placed in the public domain.

2. Distorted reporting (Jureidini et al, 2004a). Major medical journals have allowed pharmaceutical companies to publish papers in which the message (affirmations of efficacy and safety) is at odds with the reported outcomes (minimal statistical significance; dubious clinical significance). The response of The Journal of the American Academy of Child and Adolescent Psychiatry to a letter drawing attention to the shortcomings of the Keller et al. (2001) paper was interesting (Keller et al, 2001; Jureidini and Tonkin, 2003). They

declined our request that they make an editorial comment on how such distorted reporting eluded their editorial process. When we tried to press the point, the editor told us 'you have not been appointed as the guardian of the Journal, or of the profession of child and adolescent psychiatry' (letter, dated Dec 26th 2002). We remain concerned that the Keller et al. (2001) paper was allowed to be published without a clear statement to the effect that, neither paroxetine nor imipramine were statistically different to placebo on the two primary efficacy measures. The published reply to our letter also accused us of taking a position of moral superiority, and making covert claims, presumably about drug company influence. We are unclear why Keller et al. (2003) thought we were being covert in any argument (Keller et al, 2003). We overtly stated that their article misrepresented the facts collected and that the most likely reason was their bias due to industry association.

Another example of misleading reporting comes from the Wagner et al (2004) publication (Wagner et al, 2004). This paper describes a statistically significant response to Citalopram in children and adolescents on the basis of a study carried out by Lundbeck/Forest. What the authors failed to point out is that another study carried out by Lundbeck did not show an advantage of Citalopram over placebo. This study should have been mentioned in the American Journal of Psychiatry paper but was not. The negative study might never have had attracted attention had not the Committee for the Safety of Medicine already made public the fact that it existed (Committee on Safety of Medicines, 2004). Whilst the report of the positive study was accepted for publication in December 2003, it was not published until June 2004 by which time the all the authors and the journal had the capacity to know of the negative study. Either they simply failed to notice the public debate over anti-depressants in children or they turned a blind eye to it.

3. Increasing concerns about possible increased suicidal risk adverse events; and addictiveness (Medawar and Hardon, 2004). Medawar and Hardon have argued that the SSRIs are potent causes of withdrawal symptoms so it is only a matter of institutional semantics that they are not regarded as addictive. The MHRA has concluded that for all SSRI antidepressants except fluoxetine, the risks of suicide outweigh any proven benefit. The US Food and Drug Administration, after significant vacillation, have decided that SSRI drugs warrant a 'black box' warning because of the risk of suicide (FDA Public Health Advisory, 2004). The FDA's cautious conclusions about other SSRIs are not supported by a report from the American College of Neuro-psychopharmacology (American College of Neuropsychopharmacology, 2004). However the task force that wrote that report includes a number of the authors of the papers on SSRIs widely criticised in 2004. Furthermore while it is claimed that they had 'no financial support from the pharmaceutical industry', the organisation receives 'unrestricted educational grants from the

pharmaceutical industry'. This suggests that the organisation believes that if there is a degree of separation between the activity and source of funding, then the activity would be free from influence. The authors of the American College of Neuropsychopharmacology report are misguided in thinking that information about adverse effects is most likely to come from 'well designed clinical trials'. In fact history shows that major side effects undetected in clinical trials are most commonly found through what begin as anecdotal reports. As many as 51% of approved drugs have serious adverse affects not detected prior to approval (US General Accounting Office, 1990).

Patients reports of adverse drug reactions are often dismissed as unscientific, it is only the collective weight of such reports that have led to the identification of serious side effects of many drugs where randomised control have failed to reveal the dangers, such as has been the case with Paroxetine (Herxheimer and Mintzes, 2004).

Strategies for a marketing campaign

If the sceptics are right, the days may be numbered for SSRIs as block buster drugs. Nevertheless if we were running a pharmaceutical company we would not be giving up on them yet. Doctors are, after all, still prescribing high levels of Benzodiazepines in spite of clear knowledge about their addictive properties and lack of cost effectiveness. Consider the situation for executives of a drug company under pressure to increase sales of a middle ranking anti-depressant or risk losing their highly paid jobs. If we were in that situation we would still be interested in expanding into the child and adolescent market. We might begin by carrying out a large multi-centred trial of our anti-depressant in children and adolescents involving as many centres and as many psychiatrists as possible. We would have an incentive from the FDA in doing so – just researching in paediatric population entitles the company to a six month extension of patent on the anti-depressant. Our study would have as many measures as possible from the wide range quoted in the relatively small literature. We would not be put off if our study failed to show any benefit or cost effectiveness. So many people already have faith in anti-depressants that even a neutral result can lead to a statement like 'this adds a little bit to the evidence for the effectiveness of anti-depressants in children' or, 'there is no definitive evidence yet but we are confident that that is just around the corner'. We would use the study to work on opinion leaders and other psychiatrists. Professors and other senior psychiatrists would be on our advisory panel and flown to important meetings that might need to be held in Florence, New York or Paris. We would want to give the impression that they are working hard and making a solid contribution to the development of our drug but we would ensure that they had a very comfortable experience.

We would be conscious that we have more to gain from increasing the *overall* market for antidepressants in children (in tacit collaboration with competitors) rather than worrying too much about competing with them for *market share.* With illnesses like Type 1 diabetes it is possible to calculate the target population with a high degree of accuracy and this target population is limited and agreed by all parties. Thus if I want to increase my sales of my company's insulin it must be at the expense of other companies' sales. With depression the situation is different. While we will still compete one with another for market share, more of our energy will go towards increasing the overall market. A 15% share of 2 million customers is better than a 20% share of 1 million customers. We would be confident that we are nowhere near the limit of young people who can be diagnosed with depression and treated with my drug. 3 goals for market development would be:

- Increased length of treatment.
- Wider definition of depression.
- Broader indications for antidepressants (e.g., social phobia).

Part of the strategy for market expansion might be to fund and support self help groups and public health promotion projects. We would not be fussed if the front line of such projects was cognitive behavioural therapy or other non-drug interventions. We would know that most people with 'depression' are seen by GPs and others without access to CBT etc, and who would therefore be likely to prescribe, even if drugs aren't recommended as first line treatment. So all we would need to do would be to have anti-depressants recognised as *one* appropriate treatment for at least *some* children and adolescents. We would then be confident that money apparently being spent on health promotion would in fact be expanding the market for depression and therefore for our drug.

The rhetorical background to the aggressive treatment of depression usually includes references to suicide prevention. We would therefore also promote the fear that a consequence of 'ignoring depression' is suicide. Since suicide is such a rare event and so unpredictable its prevention is highly problematic.

We would be very careful that all of our published product information was cautious about the use of anti-depressants in children. Nor would we have our drug detailers explicitly promoting off label use of the drug. Rather, we would have them make statements like 'we are not allowed to recommend this for children but you make up your own mind'.

Why would we be confident that such an approach would be effective? It's not just that we run a multi-billion dollar company with an enormous marketing budget, it is also that we know that doctors and the public will collude with this exaggeration of the benefits of anti-depressants. For the medical system it is cheaper (though not more cost effective) to prescribe than to carry out other treatments for depression. Sometimes it suits families to conceptualize distress, despair and anguish as illnesses rather than looking for the meaning of such experiences.

Recommendations

1 Antidepressant drugs cannot confidently be recommended as a treatment option for childhood depression.

2 A more critical approach to ensuring the validity of published data is required.

3 Until we combine the knowledge that comes from RCTs with pharmacoepidemiological data from observational studies, we will not gain an adequate view of the benefits and harms of drug treatment (Editorial, 2004).

4 All drug trials should be registered at the time of their implementation and the details of those trials must be made available to major medical journals, so that when the papers are submitted editors have the opportunity to assess the reported data against

a. The aim set out in the initial protocol and

b. Any other as yet unpublished studies.

References

American College of Neuropsychopharmacology 2004 Preliminary Report of the Task Force on SSRIs and Suicidal Behaviour in Youth. (2004) http://www.acnp.org/exec_summary.pdf Accessed July, 2004.

Committee on Safety of Medicines, Medicines and Health Care Products Regulatory Agency. (2004) Selective Serotonin Reuptake Inhibitors (SSRIs)—overview of regulatory status and CSM advice relating to major depressive disorder (MDD) in children and adolescents: summary of clinical trials. Available at: http://medicines.mhra.gov.uk/ourwork/monitorsafequalmed/ safetymessages/ssrioverviewclintrialdata_101203.htm. Accessibility verified March 12, 2004.

Craig, J., Whittington, C.J., Kendall, T., Fonagy, P., Cottrell, D., Cotgrove, A. and Boddington, E. (2004) Selective serotonin reuptake inhibitors in childhood depression: systematic review of published versus unpublished data. *The Lancet* 363, 1341-1345.

Delate, T., Gelenberg, A.J., Simmons, V.A. and Motheral, B.R. (2004) Trends in the use of antidepressants in a national sample of commercially insured paediatric patients, 1998 to 2002. *Psychiatric Services* 55, 387 – 391

Editorial. (2004) Benefits and harms of drug treatments: Observational studies and randomised trials should learn from each other. *British Medical Journal* 329, 2-3.

Estes, R. (1996) *Tyranny of the Bottom Line: Why Corporations Make Good People do Bad Things*. San Francisco: Berrett-Koehler.

FDA Public Health Advisory October 15, 2004. Suicidality in Children and Adolescents Being Treated With Antidepressant Medications. http://www.fda.gov/cder/drug/antidepressants/SSRIPHA200410.htm Accessed November, 2004

Garland, E.J. (2004) Facing the Evidence: Antidepressant treatment in children and adolescents. *Canadian Medical Association Journal* 170, 489 – 491

Herxheimer, A. and Mintzes, B. (2004) Antidepressants and adverse effects in young patients: uncovering the evidence. *Canadian Medical Association Journal* 170, 487 – 488.

Hollinghurst, S., Kessler, D., Peters, T.J. and Gunnell, D. (2005) Opportunity cost of antidepressant prescribing in England: analysis of routine data. *British Medical Journal* 330, 999-1000

Industrial interests versus public health: the gap is growing (2004). *Prescribe International* 13, 71-76

Jureidini, J., Doecke, C., Mansfield, P., Haby, M., Menkes, D. and Tonkin, A. (2004a) Efficacy and safety of antidepressants for children and adolescents. *British Medical Journal* 328, 879-83

Jureidini, J., Tonkin, A. and Mansfield, P. (2004b) TADS study raises concerns. *British Medical Journal* 329, 1343-1344.

Jureidini, J. and Mansfield, P. (2001) Does drug promotion adversely influence doctors' abilities to make the best decisions for patients? *Australasian Psychiatry* 9, 95-100.

Jureidini, J. and Tonkin, A. (2003) Paroxetine in major depression (letter). *Journal of the American Academy of Child and Adolescent Psychiatry* 42, 514.

Keller, M.B., Ryan, N.D., Strober, M., Klein, R.G., Kutcher, S.P. and Birmaher, B. et al. (2001) Efficacy of paroxetine in the treatment of adolescent major depression: a randomized, controlled trial. *Journal of the American Academy of Child and Adolescent Psychiatry* 40, 762-72.

Keller, M.B., Ryan, N.D., Strober, M., Weller, E.B., McCafferty, J.P. and Hagino, O.R. et al. (2003) Paroxetine in major depression (letter). *Journal of the American Academy of Child and Adolescent Psychiatry* 42, 515-6.

Kondro, W. and Sibbald, B. (2004) Drug company experts advise staff to withhold data about SSRI use in children. *Canadian Medical Association Journal* 170, 783.

Medawar, C. and Hardon, A. (2004) *Medicines Out of Control? Antidepressants and the Conspiracy of Goodwill*. Amsterdam: Aksant.

Moncrieff, J. (2004) Is psychiatry for sale? An examinination of the influence of the pharmaceutical industry on academic and practical psychiatry. *A Maudsley Discussion Paper*. http://www.healthyskepticism.org/index.htm Accessed 1st July, 2004

Moynihan, R. (1998) *Too Much Medicine? The Business of Health and Its Risks for you.* Sydney: ABC Books.

National Institute for Health Care Management (NIHCM) (2002). Changing patterns of pharmaceutical innovation. **www.nihcm.org/innovations.pdf**

Orlowski, J.P. and Wateska, L. (1992) The effects of pharmaceutical firm enticements on physician prescribing patterns: There's no such thing as a free lunch. *Chest.*102, 270-73

Sagarin, B.J., Cialdini, R.B., Rice, W.E. and Serna, S.B. (2002) Dispelling the illusion of invulnerability: the motivations and mechanisms of resistance to persuasion. *Journal of Personal and Social Psychology* 83, 526-541.

SHEP Cooperative Research Group (1991). Prevention of stroke by antihypertensive drug treatment in older persons with isolated systolic hypertension. Final results of the Systolic Hypertension in the Elderly Program (SHEP). *Journal of the American Medical Association* 265, 3255-64.

Stelfox, H.T., Chua, G., O'Rourke, K. and Detsky, A.S. (1998) Conflict of interest in the debate over calcium-channel antagonists. *New England Journal of Medicine* 338, 101-106.

Treatment for Adolescents With Depression Study Team (2004). Fluoxetine, Cognitive-Behavioral Therapy, and Their Combination for Adolescents With Depression: Treatment for Adolescents With Depression Study (TADS) Randomized Controlled Trial. *Journal of the American Medical Association* 292, 807-820

US General Accounting Office. *FDA Drug Review: Postapproval Risks, 1976-85.* Washington, DC: US General Accounting Office; April 26, 1990. GAO/PEMD-90-15.

Wagner, K.D., Ambrosini, P., Rynn, M., Wohlberg, C., Yang, R. and Greenbaum, M.S., et al. (2003) Efficacy of sertraline in the treatment of children and adolescents with major depressive disorder: two randomized controlled trials. *Journal of the American Medical Association* 290, 1033-41.

Wagner, K.D., Robb, A.S., Findling, R.L., Jin, J., Guetierrez, M.M., Heydorn, W.E. (2004) A Randomised placebo-controlled trial of Citalopram for the treatment of major depression in children and adolescents. *American Journal of Psychiatry* 161, 1079–1083

Wilkes, M.S., Doblin, B.H. and Shapiro, M.F. (1992) Pharmaceutical advertisements in leading medical journals: Experts' assessments. *Annals of Internal Medicine* 116, 912-919.

Zito, J.M., Derivan, A.T. and Greenhill, L.L. (2004) Making research data available: an ethical imperative demonstrated by the SSRI debacle. *Journal of the American Academy of Child and Adolescent Psychiatry* 43, 512 – 514.

3
Culture and the Mental Health of Children: · The 'cutting edge' of expertise

Begum Maitra

"*It is tradition that changes: indeed, it is all that can.*"
(Strathern, 1992: 11)

Introduction

A gathering pile of books, journals and conference flyers bears witness to the academic interest triggered by global migrations and its effects on urban Western spaces, changing them in unpredictable ways and making them essentially multi-cultural. Despite this social and health policy lag behind, continuing to rely on theoretical concepts given shape by certainties no longer valid. It is scarcely surprising that the distinctive elements of any nation's mental health policy arise from the preoccupations of the indigenous culture. However, whether or not other cultural models are tolerated, or treated with interest as alternative ways of managing universal human concerns, varies with the host country's stand on immigrants and 'multiculturalism' (Kirmayer and Minas, 2000). The hope that immigrants would simply 'integrate' with the host culture has not been realised. Instead, immigrant groups hold on to their cultural beliefs and practices in the face of indigenous disapproval or more active opposition with an impressive tenacity (e.g. Dembour, 2001; Maitra, in press). This chapter reflects some of the debates within Western psychological and social work disciplines, both among academics and practitioners, about how multiculturalism might be put into practice. It discusses the difficulties that arise in mental health practice with children and families when insufficient attention is paid to the facts of globalisation, and the hybridised cultures that result. The chapter begins with a look at notions of expert knowledge that have arisen within Euro-American cultures, and at what experts in these cultures say about children and their relationships with family. It takes the example of 'child-centredness', central to much Western legal and social policy and which permeates international thinking on children's rights and welfare (though not without debate – see Maitra, in press). The validity of these ideas is explored through clinical examples of the cultural diversity of inner London, and consideration given to how these concepts, imbued with the authority of 'expert' knowledge, affect the lives of children and are perhaps more likely to cause harm than good.

Britain's record[1] in promoting dialogue between the indigenous and minority communities that live within her boundaries is notably distinct from that of certain other European countries, particularly from France in recent times[2] (BBC News, 2 Sep 2004). Such debates around cultural practice have, understandably, often adopted the framework of the Western discourse on rights. Minority communities argue for their 'cultural rights' and for the rights of their children to develop 'cultural identities' consonant with their ethnic groups. While these may be useful strategies for minority groups wishing to effect political change, they create particular difficulties for the clinical arena in which individual and collective interests on both sides (of professionals and of minority ethnic 'users' of clinical services) interweave in complex ways. As the clinical vignettes in the next section of this chapter will show, the real-life contexts of children may permit a wide range of solutions, often from unpredictable sources, that do not fit the simpler categories of ethnicity adopted in political and cultural rights debates.

Is expert knowledge 'culture free'?

'Despite their deficiencies, experts can be dangerous'. (Oxman et al, 2004, p 60)

It is a common experience today for a clinician to be greeted with a 'patient' (client/user) who has trawled the internet to research their problems, select their diagnosis and a preferred method of treatment. The social and political movements that have contributed to this 'democratisation of intellectual enterprise' (David Schneider, quoted in Carsten, 2000, p 2) include feminism, the civil rights movement, the rise of consumer representation and rights, and the paths these have taken within very particular Western economic, social and legal contexts. While a religious world view might continue to speak of 'knowledge' as arising from divine revelation (of truth), this is likely to be a minority view within most Western societies.

The weakening hold of 'traditional systems' of received knowledge has been accompanied by a growing suspicion of those who claim authority, expertise or other forms of elite status. However, it has left many with a yearning for

---

[1] This was not countered, but merely thrown into sharp focus, by recent debates about the relevance of 'multiculturalism' triggered by Trevor Phillips (Head of the Commission for Racial Equality) in his interview to *The Times* on 3 April 2004. He argued that citizenship demanded the 'integration' of minority groups into British culture.

[2] A law was passed in 2003 banning students at French state schools from wearing 'conspicuous' religious apparel, such as Jewish skull caps, Islamic headscarves, Sikh turbans and large Christian crosses.

alternative locations of certainty. The Western-style clinical encounter (exported widely also to the ex-colonies of Western nations) reflects these essentially contradictory drives, to individuality, autonomy and self-assertion expressed as choice, and towards its opposite. This expresses itself as a search for newer forms of authority and a reliance on modern groups based on choice (e.g. peer groups, user groups, self-help groups) rather than on traditional hierarchies (e.g. kin relationships, traditional family groups, and the clinical dyad of expert and 'patient'). This ambivalence towards 'professionalism' and 'expertise' has led in the last decade to a call for greater transparency in what experts do, and an insistence on 'evidence'. Somewhat ironically, the nature of 'evidence' itself has become more uncertain in post-modern societies as an understanding of the social construction of 'discovered' facts and systems of knowledge makes it harder to ignore the essential bias created by 'context'. Despite this undoubted cultural change in how data is thought about, it cannot·be assumed that prestigious academic teams will attempt to eliminate, or disclose, sources of bias. Major mainstream journals have raised questions about the cultural bias in research methodology (eg Boynton, Wood and Greenhalgh, 2004), and about editorial discrimination against papers from lower-income countries (Tyrer, 2005). Indeed, the need to recruit trained professionals from these very same lower-income countries signals the unstable hierarchies between nations. Recent writers also urge Western mental health experts to look for effective alternative forms of expertise from less technologically advanced nations (McKenzie, Patel and Araya, 2004).

Western folk-beliefs about the nature of knowledge and 'expertise'

A recent irreverent look at 'experts' by Oxman et al (2004) identifies common concerns that the public have about them – from hidden financial interests in what experts promote as knowledge, to the fact that the value systems of those who claim expertise often differ greatly from those affected by their opinions. This challenge to traditional sources of academic prestige and authority originating in the West has spread to those non-Western countries who have heretofore been its consumers. This development owes as much to post-colonialist and post-modern critiques of Western intellectual hegemony as to the emergence of new centres of cultural and economic influence across the globe (Hannerz, 2002; Harris, 2005).

The psychological disciplines (to which psychiatry, as a branch of medicine, sometimes bears an uneasy relationship) have much to learn from the self-reflexivity that is respectable within the social sciences (Krause, 1998; Krause, in press; Maitra, 2004a). It might seem odd that the training of mental health professionals does not require an understanding of the personal and professional[3] biases they bring to their work. The origins of this curious lack of self-awareness might lie in Western traditions of 'professionalism' that rely heavily on scientific rationality, promoting a distrust of information considered personal, subjective and emotional, and privileging those considered to be objective, logical, and rational. Carsten (2000, p 11) writes –

" . . . the fact that the science of biology itself admits no distinction between physical phenomena and the study of these phenomena marks a telling difference from social sciences such as anthropology".

In the Euro-American tradition of knowledge as something discovered rather than invented, the biological sciences claim an access to 'truth', namely, when the hidden 'facts' of nature are finally revealed. Thus what the culture perceives as a natural fact is not only part of its body of folk-beliefs, but also becomes enshrined in its intellectual traditions. As the boundaries of what is 'natural' is re-drawn by technological innovations (for example, as the new reproductive technologies re-define parenthood), greater attention becomes necessary to prevent the preoccupations of one culture, made 'natural fact' by its scientific body, from being declared as universal truths. Indeed, as the biographies of the heroes of Western science show, their discoveries are not only situated in particular historical and cultural milieus but must also be read in the context of their work practices, gendered identities, and career paths.

The shared cultural premises that underlie academic and popular concerns make it particularly difficult to identify cultural bias masquerading as expertise. This is perhaps especially tricky when attempting definitions as fundamental as those of personhood, or the nature of affectional relationships[4]. While the recursive relationships between health professionals and the public are undoubtedly valuable in helping to focus professional activities on pragmatic solutions to everyday problems, these can also obscure important and complex concepts. The drive to de-mystify professional language (by eliminating 'jargon') is welcome indeed, but allows the confusion of meanings contained within professional and 'public' uses of common English words, such as attachment, loss, counselling and 'positive input'. While a certain amount of this colloquialisation of professional ideas occurs inadvertently, through misspelling[5] and similar

---

[3] The psychodynamic schools of therapy form a notable exception to this, though few trainings include an analysis of Western cultural bias.

[4] It is here that cross-cultural material is helpful, rendering the 'invisible' culture of the observer/professional more evident through comparison with a different culture, separating what *may* be universal from what is culture-specific.

[5] For example, while agoraphobia spelt as 'aggro-phobia' may sound plausible and reassuringly familiar, it misleadingly suggests links, through the contemporary 'aggro', with ideas about stress, aggravation, and even aggression.

errors it would be a mistake to think that distortions or over-simplifications have little real impact on professional practice. For example, it is now widely accepted that behaviour problems in children may mask significant emotional difficulties, requiring skilled psychological intervention ('treatment') rather than the increase of discipline, or affection, alone. The common simplification of 'skilled psychological intervention' into 'support' may be dismissed as an understandable attempt to de-stigmatise 'mental health'[6] matters, but blurs the crucial distinction between 'ordinary' distress that might benefit from affection and practical support, and the more serious implications of 'disorder'.

The Western family

'Family' talk in contemporary Western contexts

"Our understandings of the nature of the child are too varying over time and too related to contemporary intellectual ambience to permit any confident conclusions about 'the child'." (Super and Harkness, 1986, p 550)

The history of ideas about the 'family' in Euro-American cultures suggests that there has been much change in recent times. Simpson (1997) argues that any representation of the family is a highly selective repertoire of normative images shaped by the reigning social forces of the day, and that it does not reflect the diversity of family forms even within that society. He suggests (*ibid.*, p 52) that Thatcherite rhetoric reified a particular vision of the family in Britain – the nuclear, heterosexual, co-resident, stable, monogamous family – as a natural, universal and self-evident structure, and that it did so as part of a project to dismantle civic and public culture. The individual and the family thus came to define the locus of enterprise, choice and consumption. This *hegemonic familism*, Simpson continues, socialises Western children to expect a particular sequence of life-events – romance, courtship, marriage, home-making and parenthood – as 'normal family life', the pattern being reinforced by the church, the media, and the legal and social systems of the welfare state. Its privacy intensified[7], 'home' becomes the physical and emotional setting for people's personal and private lives (James, 1998) and the locus for a *self* that is itself located in the family group. Referring to anxieties about the decline of the family in recent times, Strathern (1992) suggests that while the ideal of family life remains, the greater fragmentation of families is a feature

---

[6] A phrase that more often refers to its opposite, ie mental illness.

[7] Since the changing economy had altered the locus of work (as in the factory system) from within the home (as in a cottage industry system) to outside it.

of the diversity of familial lifestyles now visible. This, she notes, is a diversity based on the exercise of individual choice and the radical effects of technological and cultural change in the West. Reproductive technologies, gene therapies, gay and lesbian 'family' forms and parenthood, and the highly politicised debates about 'consumerism' in the arena of reproduction and family have resulted in a new conceptualisation of nature. Nature has been 'enterprised-up', and what was taken to be natural has become *a matter of choice.*

Through the narratives of two white, working class British individuals describing the break-up of family following divorce, Simpson (1997, p 65) explores the " . . . major fault-line between the collective pull of kinship obligation and dependency on the one hand and the drive towards individuality, independence and self-determination on the other". The latter tendency, he points out, may have as much to do with the commoditisation of intimate relationships arising out of the enterprise culture, as with self-realisation. Reinforced by individualism and consumerism, the demands for autonomy and authentic individuality make the exercise of choice nothing less than a moral imperative in contemporary Western cultures. It must be remembered that other threads of Western culture do not disappear altogether. For example, the lingering influences of a remembered morality may promote renunciation of choice and certain types of dependency[8] rather than autonomy.

Western childhoods

Critiques, arising within the Western social sciences over several decades, have pointed to the ethnocentrism of Western theories about childhood (Kessel and Siegel, 1983; Kessen, 1983) and child development (Prout, 2005), and yet have had curiously little impact on health policy and practice. The tenacity of these theories may be understood by an exploration of the 'intellectual ambience' within which Western ideas of children have developed.

Western[9] developmental psychology has grown out of the traditions of experimental (scientific) method – a logical-positivist, laboratory-based enterprise dedicated to the study of individuals. Apart from a consideration of the effects of external 'stimuli' that impinge on the individual, it has largely excluded the

---

[8] Simpson (*ibid*) cites the continuing force of ideas arising from the Christian marriage vows – "for better or for worse, in sickness and in health'.

[9] To the apparently rhetorical (or frankly impolite) 'are there other (non-Western) developmental psychologies?' the answer, of course, would be in the affirmative. Every culture constructs a system of ideas about the nature of children, the sequence of developmental stages, and the reasons things go wrong, but does so using paradigms and realms of experience that may be unfamiliar, and therefore unrecognisable, to the Western eye and ear.

environment,. An abundance of anthropological data shows that other cultures do not support the assumptions about growth and development made by Western developmental psychology. Alternate systems of belief may, of course, be equally tenacious because of being inter-linked with local networks of ideas about shared material and social circumstances. Dasen (2003) discusses a number of theoretical frameworks that show how cultural and contextual data about the lives and experiences of children contribute to a locally constructed developmental psychology. Super and Harkness (1986) propose the idea of the 'developmental niche'. Lying at the juncture of the theoretical concerns of psychology and anthropology it includes three major subsystems – the physical and social settings in which the child lives, culturally regulated customs of child care, and the psychology of the child's caretakers. It is the interaction of these that determines the nature and the timing of skills required for 'development' in a particular setting.

While Ariés' (1963) work is perhaps best known, along with other writers (such as Liljestrom, 1983; Archard, 1993; Donzelot, 1997) this body of work traces the history of the relationships between the Western state, the market system and the private sphere of the family and home. Most importantly, it tracks how these have contributed to definitions of childhood within Western societies. Liljestrom (1983) refers to the rapid growth of the public services sector in the 1960s to become the dominant source of employment for both men and women. This led to a spiralling increase in the production of 'public goods' (i.e. the produce of civil servants, doctors, nurse, psychologists, and such others) and, by removing mothers into the labour force, weakened household resources for the provision of informal child care. That this sequence of events fuelled the demand for professional child-care is not surprising, making it an essential part of the design of the Welfare State, but it also created a cultural bias that argued that children's potential was best developed by trained professionals. Parents were no longer considered 'naturally' able to perform these tasks, but needed to be equipped for these by professionals. Rather more problematically this 'local' Western trend influenced academic beliefs about child development and promoted them as universal ideas that were based on local interests. Claims made on the behalf of children, and couched in the universalising language of 'needs' as material that all children everywhere have a 'right' to (such as specially created toys for the child's 'stimulation', or particular verbal expressions of praise for the development of its 'self-esteem'), now seem unassailably right.

So self-evident do these Western theories about children seem today that to enquire into the nature and validity of these claims is likely to be seen as an assault on the authority of 'modern' scientific institutions. When these critiques are mounted by cultural minorities they appear as dangerous forms of 'traditionalism', promoting the vested interests of dominant individuals over others (usually women and children). The introduction of cultural critiques into professional debates also sparks a fear of unbridled cultural relativism, and that it will invite mainstream professionals to shirk their collective (and presumably culture-free) responsibility to the oppressed or vulnerable of any culture (Maitra, in press). However, as several writers (Archard, 1993; Donzelot, 1997) warn, the professionalized model of Western child-care defines norms of familial 'health' in such a way as to allow the subtle and pervasive intrusion of experts such as doctors, psychiatrists, lawyers and social workers, into the 'privacy' of family life. By doing so it facilitates 'the policing of families' from within.

Childhood, in (Western) scientific discourse, is characterised by change and movement, children being thought to pass through clearly defined developmental phases. The particular significance of their socialisation for the future of a society has been noted since the seventeenth century and children have been considered to need a caring control

> "... lest their potential for change run wild and their adulthood, and hence future adult society, be endangered. . . . In this way the social institution of 'childhood' – that complex of material, social, moral and economic constraints that shapes children's everyday lives – is held to place an important steadying hand upon a child's demands for access to the adult social world." (James, 1998: 141)

This responsibility to socialise the child presented it as increasingly dependent on the family and the home. By the nineteenth century, a mass of child protection legislation was required to safeguard children from irresponsible carers and unsuitable homes. The late twentieth century has seen further changes in the status of children. Along with extension of the social institution of childhood (to 19 or 21 years, into the phase of 'young person'-hood), acknowledgement of children's rights and of their capacity as independent social actors, there are also increasing legal and economic constraints on their independence.

> "More generally 'childhood' has become the focus for a range of often contradictory ethical and political debates, so that what may be regarded as one person's independent child may be another's evidence of neglect; what might be seen as familial care may be experienced by the child as familial control." (James, ibid.: 145)

Parenting and cultural attitudes towards dependency

Let us consider the combined effects on 'parenting' of the following – the professionalisation of childcare (and a parallel notion of parents as amateurs), the re-definitions of nature by technology (taking the bearing and rearing of

children out of the 'natural' and into the realm of 'expertise'), and the
ambivalence towards 'traditional' notions of marriage and parenthood
introduced by the growing emphasis on individual choice and by the diversity
of life-style choices. Liljestrom (1983) writes about Danish parents' insecurity
about how they should rear their children, and of their perceptions of the
difficulties of child rearing. She points to the widespread reluctance among
parents to influence their children, originating in a cultural belief that it was
wrong[10] to influence people. "*The seeds of liberalism and free upbringing*" she
notes "*have grown into plants of timidity and insecurity.*" (Liljestrom, *ibid.*:
141). This erosion of parental confidence confounds the very hopes and wishes
that may have prompted these individuals to become parents. The sense of
competition with professionals, promoted as the only source of expert
understanding for their children, leaves many parents feeling cheated of their
entitlement to the emotional satisfactions of parenting – such as intimacy,
parental self-esteem, and the child's trust and love. It can sometimes result in
parents turning over the 'impossible' task of rearing their child to professionals.

In a more recent study of British teachers at a primary school James
(1998) describes how everyday understandings of the child and of what
childhood should be influences teachers' perceptions of their pupils. The
school was situated in a 'mixed neighbourhood' and the staff members were
reported to feel some concern at the increasingly working-class profile of the
pupils. A home visit was routinely conducted before the children started at
school, and in an acerbic tone James comments (*ibid.*, p 148) on the 'rhetoric
of concern' that saw this as 'beneficial'. The teachers' images of childhood
were based on assumptions about "*a carefree mythical childhood*", and about
"*what a* child *should be: happy in an innocent and dependent vulnerability*"
(*ibid.*, p 154). Their understanding of these particular children assumed a
fairly direct correspondence between the social and economic circumstances
of the home and the academic potential of the child, and were effectively
based on stereotypes routinely depicted in the media. The teachers read the
physical state of the home for signs of parenting skills, inferring from this the
kinds of socialising experiences the child was receiving. The child's behaviour
and potential were read as simply the dependent and passive outcomes of its
nurturing background. As the child's relationship with the teacher developed
over time these opinions were modified. The staff members were reportedly
always eager to retain some hope in a child's potential for change and
betterment, but tended to continue attributing weaknesses in the child's
achievements or behaviour to the contexts of home and family. Reasons for
failure were located 'within' the child only as a last resort, and only after some

---

[10] The same culturally based tentativeness presented by British parents towards their
children is described, albeit in a more light-hearted vein, by a general practitioner
(Tristan, 2005).

time had elapsed. Explanations for academic success, rather interestingly, focussed upon the child-teacher relationship!

Through their liaison work with schools mental health clinicians are likely to be familiar with how popular notions influence teachers' perceptions of children and their families. Yet it may be more difficult to identify where these same popular notions creep into their own clinical practice. Such influence may be explicitly dressed up as professional preferences for particular research or theoretical propositions, but more covertly expressed in their subjective responses to their clients. Cultural 'common sense' presented as self-evident truth requires little debate, is difficult to identify and, as a result, resistant to critical scrutiny. These difficulties are made yet more obscure by a number of factors – first, the fact that the psychological disciplines share a language with a public fed a mixed diet of popular and scientific information and mis-information, making it difficult to separate professional from everyday meanings (for e.g. of words such as 'attachment', 'conflict', 'trauma'). Second, concern about the increasing influence of service-users makes it less likely that professionals will state their opinions openly, especially those that seem 'negative' or critical. These are usually driven underground by the demands of 'political correctness' or fear of complaint. James (1998) inferred teachers' hostile attitudes towards families through qualitative features such as the tone of voice, facial expression, and sarcasm, noting that exaggeration and metaphor often indicated value judgements.

"It is noticeable that approval was rarely voiced. The teachers were on the look-out for danger signs, . . . Thus, . . . , explanations for educational failure were more readily sought in the inadequacies of the home, than through the more uncomfortable and possibly disquieting process of reflecting on their own practice as teachers." (James, ibid.: 153, fn 10).

While both parents and professionals are likely to respond unsympathetically, even with covert harshness, when faced with children whose behaviour they cannot control or do not understand, the effects of unexamined professional bias raises worrying questions about the covert exercise of power through inappropriate pathologising (Timimi, 2005). These professional difficulties are especially likely when different cultural goals of socialisation make both the child's and the family's behaviour incomprehensible.

A black African teacher's repeated complaint about a 5 year old Asian boy seemed unusually harsh given his age, and curious, given her inability to say more than that his 'behaviour' was 'challenging' and 'disrespectful'. It was only after much discussion by the psychologist of the elusiveness of cultural meanings that the teacher blurted out her belief that the child was 'sexist', and that this was part of his 'socialisation by his culture'. Further exploration identified the event that appeared to be the source of this belief. On one occasion while the child's mother had been tearfully confiding in the teacher about domestic difficulties, the teacher had noted with some outrage that the child appeared to be 'laughing'. Subsequent discussion with the teacher ranged across a number of areas, such as – how inferences are drawn from observations of emotion in children, and distinctions made between derisory laughter and other states (such as anxious grimacing or laughter); how cultural models influence emotional expression, and vary with region, class and private/public domains; the cognitive and emotional capacities of 5 year olds (to grasp, empathise with and react to adult emotion, particularly that of a significant adult); the cross-cutting influences of attachment to a primary carer (e.g. the mother) and the induction of boys into gendered hierarchies. Also crucial to this process was the exploration of the particular features of the teacher's own history and socialisation, and the effects of these on her expectations of children, and their relationships with their mothers.

How can the apparent lack of sympathy among professionals for the experiences of children (in the clinical vignette) or for their families (as in the study by James discussed above) be understood? A clue may be found in observations made by Prof Aynsley-Green (2003, p 4-5) –

"I argue there is something very peculiar about how we in the UK and England, in particular, view children compared to, for example, Sweden, Finland, Spain, Italy and Portugal. There is something very strange about our coldness towards children and the lack of value we attach to them and to childhood." and

" . . . childhood as we have known it, is disappearing. Disappearing because of relentless commercialisation of children, relentless sexualisation of children and the loss of time for children to be children, to learn to gain the skills to be competent adults." (underlining mine)

The history of childhood in the West suggests the increasing portrayal of children as dependent, demanding and requiring an extraordinarily high level of 'expert' attention. The resulting obligation to provide care poses an area of conflict with other dominant cultural expectations, namely, the drive to autonomy and the expectation that one will be free to pursue individual self-fulfilment. This tension is likely to create an ambivalence, albeit unconscious, towards dependent individuals. This is not to say that cultures which promote collective rather than individual goals are untroubled by similar feelings, but rather that the balance of obligations towards oneself and dependent others is weighted by a congruent system of rewards and sanctions. Thus, individuals in some non-Western cultures are socialised into feeling increased self-worth, and expecting the approval of others, when individual needs are sacrificed in favour of another's, and to feeling shame and guilt when these ideals are not met. Contemporary language in Western settings rarely speaks of sacrifice[11] as an ideal, and more commonly promotes self-worth as being achievable through self-expression (of 'inner' states and feelings), choice and its expression through self-assertion.

The demands of child care (as also the care of other dependents, such as the elderly or disabled) are likely to regularly interrupt adult self-expression and to provoke intense ambivalence. Unleavened by the social rewards available in many non-Western cultures, such as the high status accorded to motherhood and the close networks of kinswomen or domestic assistants, there is a need to find an alternative focus for this ambivalence towards children, and the guilt engendered by it. The intensity of contemporary preoccupations with 'perpetrators' of harm to children suggests where this displacement may have led. Importantly, a focus on individual 'perpetrators' of injustice or oppression permits complacency about the collective responsibility of the larger group (as Prof Aynsley-Green suggests) for environments that permit, if not tacitly condone, other forms of harm. Its counterpart may be found in the urge to allocate responsibility to other collective bodies, such as to professional, political, or national groups[12] outside one's own. Admittedly, the advantage of distance perhaps allows a clearer view of how alien collective beliefs lead to abuses of power. The apparent tone of sympathy when attributing risks to children to states of 'disadvantage' (in certain groups or nations) is misleading, and also insufficient in itself as an explanation for all the risks that children may face. Continuing inequities in distributions of wealth, both within affluent nations and across nations, lends little confidence in collective commitments to eradicating even those risks arising directly from economic disadvantage, and call into question the intention of governments towards those who are most vulnerable, namely children[13]. Current governmental rhetoric in the United Kingdom to promote the 'inclusion' of disadvantaged children fails to reassure, and concerns have been voiced that small packages of resources (Coote et al, 2004) scattered across the public and voluntary sectors may do little more than salve the collective conscience.

---

[11] While altruism remains a valued ideal, it is perhaps least conflicted when focussed on a distant recipient (such as drought victims in Africa), and does not obstruct self-expression.

[12] It permits an extrusion of one's worst fears about the failures of one's own group.

[13] Shiva Kumar (1998) argues that the 'welfare approach' stigmatises the most disadvantaged (chiefly women and children everywhere) as recipients of charity. A framework of human rights rather than welfare would ensure that states took responsibility to provide for the essential needs of children.

Contemporary childhoods – Globalisation, consumerism and multicultural spaces

To a greater or lesser degree, the project of the self becomes translated into one of the possession of desired goods and the pursuit of artificially framed styles of life. (. . .) Not just lifestyles, but self-actualisation is packaged and distributed according to market criteria.   Giddens, (1991: 198)

Cultural heterogeneity is hard to eradicate through legislation. While the intentions that lay behind the recent French ban (discussed above) on public markers of religious identities have been vigorously debated, it is nevertheless unlikely to promote cultural homogeneity or integration. Indeed, the variety and intensity of opinions it continues to provoke may be said to maintain the focus on cultural difference. The small numbers of minority ethnic individuals in European countries and in Britain do not explain the volume and rate of cultural exchange in these countries. It is necessary to acknowledge the unavoidable flow of ideas that trade and tourism inevitably engender, adding to the constant stream of global migrations. These ideas contain within them the remnants of, and counter-responses to, old relationships of power between nations. Hannerz (2002) points out that the cultural centres of the world today are not necessarily the same as those that wield economic and military power. Contemporary 'cultural flows' may follow unexpected trajectories, from the 'periphery' to the 'centre' (as from Islamic countries in the Middle East to Islamic populations in the West), or to another 'peripheral' locus (as in the impact of Indian film on North and West Africa).

Postcolonial theorists have argued that projections of the other are also always about repressed aspects of the self. Hall (1996) discusses the centuries old sense of white superiority over racialised others, and the difficulty of Western nations in accommodating to being *"only a minor player in the great affairs of the globe"* (p 67). She comments on the British Labour Party's reluctance to discard notions of a homogenous nation state, and that it has the paradoxical effect of provoking cultural nationalisms (such as among Islamic and some black groups). Cultural consumerism provides another solution to this reduced sense of self, notable in the appetite for a diversity of instant 'identities' and the exaggerated sense of entitled access to these that global markets and tourism permit[14]. As the two vignettes below show, this traffic of cultural

---

[14] While the liberal Western professional classes may revel in the multiplicity of choices, of following an *Ayurvedic* massage with a Japanese meal and an evening of *salsa* dancing, there is a risk of mistaking such access as 'understanding'. While any route to relief of discomfort may seem worth considering, whether through easy cross-cultural borrowings or more committed study, the risk is that partial and 'trivialised' (through fragmentation, inadequate translation, and incommensurate categories) accounts of meaning may be mistaken for the whole.

symbols in Western urban centres makes for an unpredictability in children's experiences, and for a greater and more confusing diversity than professional frameworks for self, individuality or identity currently accommodate.

A young white Briton had converted to the religion of the South Asian population she had lived among since her birth in a city in northern England. She spoke the language as well as her peers (second generation South Asians), and was deeply steeped in their cultural customs. All her three partners had been South Asian, and she had brought up her children, who were barely distinguishable in appearance from other South Asian children, to think of themselves as British South Asians. When difficulties arose with her management of her considerable parental responsibilities it was her cultural 'conversion' that was considered most suspect, and cited most commonly by professionals as evidence of possible disorder (notably, of immature or 'border-line' personality).

A West African 13 year old girl spoke longingly of wanting straight black hair like that of the Indian women she saw on 'Bollywood'[15] videos every night. While she spoke also of the rivalries between black and Asian girls in her East London school, the raised visibility of South Asian 'models' of achievement (in national school results, and in the unabashed appeal that South Asian film held for her peers across ethnic groups), a positive regard for her therapist (also South Asian), and public discourses that represented several non-White minority groups under the umbrella of 'black British', permitted a flexibility across 'ethnic' boundaries and the possibility of transfers of 'desirable' attributes, expectations and satisfactions. It must be borne in mind that the history of South Asians within the African continent, inflected through the presence of European colonisation, had created more problematic relationships between these two groups.

The cutting edge of expertise

'Child centred' practice

Prout (2005) draws attention to the changed Western image of children in the late twentieth century, and that children are more likely to be represented as active, knowledgeable, and socially participative, than as innocent, ignorant and biddable. They are therefore more difficult to manage, more troublesome and troubling. Health and legal discourse often speak of this as the dilemma of balancing care with control. Quite appropriately, rather than prescribing good practice legislation addresses the boundaries of acceptable practice,

---

[15] This refers to the prolific and popular Indian film industry based in Bombay (now Mumbai). While it began as a self-ironising reference to the Hollywood industry by Indians, Bollywood may now legitimately claim a sizeable influence in many non-Western countries (Larkin, 2002).

requiring action to minimise risk in situations in which the child's interests might be overlooked. However, what may be 'good practice' across all socio-cultural categories and contexts remains difficult to define. This is in part due to the lack of agreement about what is in the 'best interests' of children. These concepts appear to point agreeably to a consensus that might, in time, be reached by all those who aspire to build 'child-centred' societies. Nonetheless, there is more than a touch of circularity in this way of thinking. Developmental 'needs' allocated to children by (more affluent) societies self-designated as 'child-centred', are reified by the same cultural bias within their academic bodies. Now framed as 'rights', these may lay claim to 'universal' validity resting on the hegemonic claims of the society espousing them (Boyden, 1997). However, as Prout (*ibid.*) points out, declarations such as the United Nations Convention of the Rights of the Child have been described as high in rhetoric and lofty principle, but about which little needs to be done in practice.

If, as seems to be indicated by the wealth of ethnographic data from non-Western cultures (eg Das, 2003; Saraswathi, 2003; Le Vine et al, 1996; Nsamenang, 1992; Rogoff et al, 1975; Whiting and Whiting, 1975), notions of children and their needs have not been universally formulated in similar ways, how does Western psychological theory attempt to address this diversity? I have discussed elsewhere (Maitra, 1995; 1996; 2004b) the costs to minority ethnic children, and their families, of continuing cultural incompetence among professionals. However, there is a more fundamental problem about the rigidity of existing professional beliefs which are based on an insistence on Western paradigms of what it is to be 'human', in other words, on an outdated imperialism.

A South Asian teenager, under treatment for what was presumed to be a serious mental illness, was picked up late at night by the police, wandering in a state of apparent confusion. His parents' inadequate awareness of the risks to him suggested to the police that they were insufficiently concerned about him, and therefore unable to supervise him, and he was not returned home. The father, an elderly man who suffered from a physical illness which required complex routines of treatment and monitoring, was unable to give an adequate account of his son's activities and whereabouts before his disappearance from home. When pressed to acknowledge the (genuine) risks to his son of wandering alone while under heavy medication the father grew increasingly agitated, and objected vehemently to being accused of being an inadequate father. His wife's absence at successive meetings was explained somewhat vaguely by statements that she was unwell or asleep. Eventually, the father burst out in anger and distress "I must look after myself, or I will die. God will look after my son, and will do what He wills."

Caution is essential when referring to likely internal states (emotional or physical) within the father. The words selected by an observer to describe the emotional tone of the behaviour or what is said by an individual are likely to suggest more than is known with certainty, inviting premature 'closure' before adequate data is available. This tendency is heightened when disagreement or conflict are imminent, and the natural response is to prioritise one's own interests (safety, status, certainty) when 'reading' the other's intentions, rather than to question the possible sources of bias (old prejudices, fears) in ourselves. While this self-centredness may seem justifiable when serious physical risk is involved, it is more problematic when what is at stake is merely one's self-esteem (confidence in one's judgement, professional skill and the esteem of others) or professional authority[16].

Let us consider briefly the current notions of parental rights and responsibilities. Archard (1993) argues that both the right to bear children, and the right to rear them as one chooses, are not unconditional. The child's right to be reared by those who are 'best suited' is more significant than the 'blood tie'. Parents may often also be best suited *because* the blood tie is most likely to create the ties of 'bonding' that, Archard describes (with more than a touch of sentimentality), are manifest in the *"strong, self-sacrificial affection"* for their child that motivates the parent to fit the role of best possible caregiver (*ibid.*: 102-3). This notion of self-sacrificial love, akin to the ideal of 'unconditional' love, appears to promise the total prioritisation of the child above all other considerations – at least above the parent's own self-interest. By implication, such bonding occurs irrespective of other considerations, such as the particular nature of the child and the parent's response to this, and rules out also the possibility that other demands on the parent, made by family obligations, duty, honour or love, may be equally significant. While there is some animal data on increased maternal aggression (sometimes in the service of her young) due to hormonal activity during the post partum and lactating phases, there is little support for simple generalisations about human parental (or even maternal) affection and motivations. Indeed, contemporary accounts emphasise the inter-actional nature of the child-carer relationship. The importance of expectations and 'goodness of fit' between the particular natures of each have a great deal to do in predicting both short and longer-term outcomes for the child. Equally, culture and social structure dictate a variety of different orientations to the nature and obligations of the parent towards the child. Lau (1984) describes the obligation to one's parents in Chinese culture that may countenance, if not require, the sacrifice of the interests of one's child in order to save one's parent. The literature from South America and South Asia on forms of infanticide demonstrates the complexity of parental motivations even under such extreme conditions, and

---

[16] The responsibility of professionals to be cautious in their claims to expertise is indicated by a recent debate between the courts and the General Medical Council about the appropriate punishment for a senior medical professional who had based serious conclusions on grossly inadequate evidence (Dyer, 2004).

the socio-cultural concepts that make such acts comprehensible and bearable (Scheper-Hughes, 1987; 2003). It seems likely that 'self-sacrifice' and the unconditional nature of parental love might be ideals that are held across a wide enough variety of cultures to be considered universal. However, the fact that each culture is likely to interpret the underlying constructs (of self, sacrifice, love, etc) differently ensures that these ideals will not be regularly and predictably manifest in action. Furthermore, when an ideal such as parental love is promoted above others with an especial urgency it is necessary to consider other, more ambiguous, underlying motivations. Referring to the Freudian idea of *reaction-formation* (Freud, 1973:123) one might propose that a society's ambivalence towards dependency may be manifest in both the compensatory inflation of demands on behalf of children, and an over-zealousness in prescriptions for their defence. This ambivalence is also likely to be manifest in the consistent failure to address longstanding inadequacies of practice, and a deflection of responsibility to other arenas. Noting that childhood mortality rates in the United States were higher than in many poorer countries, Shiva Kumar (1998) reports a clear mismatch between national income levels and the mortality rates for children under five years (U5MR).

Let us consider another example of a father's perceptions of the limits of his parental obligations.

A working class white British father was apparently much angrier (than the father referred to above) as judged by his facial expression, loud tones and general demeanour. He threatened to throw his 11 year old son out of the house, or to beat him, if the (health) professional did not immediately arrange alternative social services accommodation. This father, having looked after his four children single-handedly following their mother's sudden death several years ago, had for some time been declaring his 'inability to cope', but with little response from services.

While both fathers (the white British and South Asian) might have been saying similar things about the limits of self-sacrifice, the culturally consonant language of the second aroused less professional concern (or criticism). The British father's threat to beat his child was correctly understood to be rhetorical, his emotional style being familiar through professional experience of the common repertoires of working-class white British men. His wish to have his son removed from his care to an alternative place was 'recognisable' as a response to the stress of parenting, and as lying within his society's available options for handing over parental responsibility (even if temporarily).

Why did the South Asian father's account (and emotional responses) fail to signal the same considerations? First, because this father appeared not to see professional agencies as partners that he might persuade (or threaten) into sharing his parental burdens. Second, because he appeared, in his brief exchange with the police, to prioritise his own health above possible risks to his son. What a South Asian man feels is 'speakable' (conscious and unconscious emotions, e.g. hurt pride, fears – for his own health, of criminal charges), when, why (as defence, as deflection, as a plea for help) and to whom, is dependent on a range of cross-cutting cultural systems that include notions of gender, of authority based on age and status, and the history of relationships with the indigenous community and its institutions. Third, because explicit reference to religious belief is uncommon in everyday talk among most Britons, and talk of divine will is more likely to be interpreted as ironic, or as flagrant evasion of individual responsibility. To cite divine authority as a real arbiter of everyday actions and consequences, and as legitimately placed above secular structures and collective formulations (of 'appropriate' emotional and social responses as in the case of the second father), is culturally incongruous in the British context and invites the application of negative meanings of one sort or another.

Cultural styles of relatedness

Cross-cultural data about parenting styles suggest that these vary greatly in accordance with the socio-cultural orientations promoted by that culture. Different styles of parenting are thought to promote different foundations for the self, for a sense of agency and of interpersonal relatedness (Kagitçibasi, 1996; Yamada, 2004). A brief summary of the links between social contexts and corresponding patterns of *independence, interdependence* or *autonomous relatedness* in children by Kagitçibasi (*ibid.*) proposes that the *independent* self is adaptive in Western, urban, educated middle-class families. Defined as an individual agent, it is bounded, self-contained, unique and separate from others. The *interdependent* self, adaptive in rural contexts with a lower socioeconomic and educational profile, is a communal agent which is basically interconnected with others, compliant and role oriented. It sees agency as externally regulated. The *autonomous-relational* self, adaptive in urban, educated, middle-class families in traditionally interdependent societies, is autonomous with respect to agency and related with respect to interpersonal distance.

Keller *et al* (2004) explore the relationships between parenting styles and the development of a particular sense of self that is concordant with the group's needs. In a comparative study of early parenting in three culturally diverse groups they explored the development of self-regulation and self-recognition in toddlers. The *proximal* parenting style emphasised close body contact with the mother, her bodily rhythms communicating to the baby a sense of fusion and synchrony. Commoner in cultures which promote interdependence and where children are needed as early as possible to work cooperatively with their families, this style fostered early self-regulation and, through bodily stimulation, promoted accelerated motor development. Keller *et al* noted the overlapping vocalisations of these mothers with their babies, and its difference from the quasidialogic vocal patterns of Euro-American mothers. The latter group's *distal* parenting style has a greater emphasis on face-to-face exchange and object stimulation. Common among independence promoting cultures this pattern emphasises eye contact and looking, reinforcing separateness and reciprocity. The use of objects and toys supports the infant's capacity to spend time alone, and fosters curiosity and exploration in the outer world. Each of these promote the development of a sense of a distinct self, and earlier development of self-recognition. The *combined* proximal and distal style of parents in autonomous-relational cultures produced self-regulation and self-recognition at intermediate levels when compared with the other two groups. It is important to emphasise that the independent and interdependent dimensions are not mutually exclusive, and that every culture negotiates between the two with the autonomous-relational type indicating intermediate positions.

It must be borne in mind that these studies identify the mechanisms through which culture influences child development by comparing parenting in more or less culturally homogenous societies. Children who grow up in the flux of multicultural urban Western communities experience a more complex interplay of several cultures that, depending on the relative positions of the indigenous and minority ethnic communities, carry more or less influence and prestige. Thus, children are likely to acquire a mix of skills that have an uncertain relevance to their immediate contexts, and are differentially valued by their peers, the ethnic community and the diversity of contexts presented by the school, the mainstream culture, and the mental health team.

A Turkish adolescent girl admitted to hospital in an acutely psychotic state, gave an account of 'gang rape' while under the influence of illegal drugs. While her parents anxiously asked to be part of the discussion with professional agencies, the girl's reluctance to include them dictated the setting up of 'individual therapy' sessions for her. A small number of 'psycho-education' sessions were offered to her parents and focused on the nature and management of their daughter's psychotic illness. The content of the girl's sessions suggested that she enjoyed discussing make-up, boys, drug use and dating with her young, white English therapist. Her belief that it would not have been possible to broach these subjects if her parents had been present was not explored, the therapist appearing to share the girl's expectation. This professional bias was likely to have been based on cultural stereotypes of 'traditional' patriarchal cultures and the expectation that immigrant parents would be rigidly opposed to certain forms of adolescent experimentation. These ideas about the harshly repressive attitudes of the minority community towards the young are often magnified by images and representations of 'culture conflict' in the media.

Little is known about how these parents knew of their daughter's activities, nor about how they felt about dating or substance abuse. However, they had clearly not prevented their daughter from dressing like her British peers or participating in their social activities. They had been told that she had been raped. When she 'chose' to press charges against her attackers they accompanied her to meetings with the police though they were unable to participate actively as they spoke little English. The girl's age and cognitive development suggested that she had the capacity to consent to treatment, and to choose not to share information with her parents. While many professional decisions were based on her 'choices', some question remained about whether this young girl was discriminating between various options available to her, or merely complying with the professional expectation that she made choices. Socialised into an expectation of interdependence, it might be argued that she was guided by a desire to gain acceptance through compliance, rather than by notions of individual, autonomous interests. While the first steps in any aspiration to autonomy might well present (as contemporary Western accounts of adolescence emphasise) in the challenge/breaking of parental rules, cultures that promote autonomy are likely to do so through a large number of varied and graded scenarios, starting early in life. These provide the child with opportunities to practice weighing up the risks and benefits of different degrees of autonomy and choice and resulting, by adolescence, in a more discerning alertness to risks. Attitudes among immigrant parents vary depending on their access to, and participation in, mainstream culture. However, they are likely, even if partially and unknowingly, to socialise their children into patterns of compliance and interdependence appropriate to their cultures of origin. This equips their children poorly for the 'choices' presented to them, and dangerously confuses genuinely autonomous choice with compliance with peers[17], or mainstream cultural choices.

The professional decision in this case to privilege the girl's choices did not question whether her age and cognitive development were adequate markers of a capacity to make choices, especially when these lay outside the cultural repertoires she had been socialised into. Professional decision-making assumed also that other notions of 'individual' rights arising from independence-promoting individualistic Western cultures (such as, the legal notion of capacity to consent exercised here as the right to refuse parental involvement) were relevant to her, and would enhance the expression of her autonomous self. The hybrid cultural socialisations of minority ethnic children, especially those born in Britain, are often underestimated because the external markers of dress, manner and language suggest that they are culturally British. Furthermore, the decisions not to explore immigrant parents' attitudes and their understanding of the risks that accompany the contemporary choices their children may make, are also likely to have been based on assumptions that the interdependent style of 'collective' cultures is repressive and harmful to children. An unquestioning and simplistic professional commitment to individualism risks losing sight of the real needs of all children and young people, for longer periods of graded dependence on trusted adults. Indeed

---

[17] These are sometimes referred to as 'family pressure' and 'peer pressure' respectively.

research indicates that adolescents in Western cultures may value degrees of continuing interdependence with adults (Offer et al, 1984; Steinberg, 1990; Hill, 1993) as they develop peer relationships and autonomy. The mistaken emphasis on autonomy in this case contributed to a loss of important opportunities to bridge important gaps of experience and understanding between the young person and her family. This may have facilitated a gradual development of more meaningful exercise of 'choice', allowing her to find intermediate positions possible between autonomy and relatedness that neither her parents nor professionals might have anticipated.

An English mother accompanied her teenage daughter for a first appointment to a child mental health clinic, with a request for 'counselling' to address the girl's feelings about a recent sexual assault. The mother prepared to wait while her daughter met with the professional, and when invited by the professional to join them she turned to the girl to ask whether she would like that. Her daughter nodded silently. Mother and daughter wept through much of the first session but made no move to offer/request comfort of each other. Despite this, their manner of speaking, tones of voice and opinions of each other suggested a very close and loving relationship. They also appeared to share a view of the assault as a traumatic event that should appropriately prompt sympathy and 'support' for both the girl and her mother, and that legal action would help achieve 'closure', allowing them to 'get on with their lives'. In later sessions that she attended on her own the girl seemed preoccupied with the following questions – what part of her (whether her body, her reputation, the 'normal' course of her life, her capacity to trust boys) had been most harmed, and to what degree; whether her wish to press charges against her attacker amounted to causing him harm (as suggested by friends they had in common); confusion and anger caused by her mother's wish to limit who she confided in about these experiences and concern that her mother thought she was 'making too much of a fuss'.

This vignette emphasises the degree to which the rights to autonomy and the expression of choice remain contested between individuals, even within Euro-American cultures. This family belonged to the upwardly mobile urban working class, and their attitudes to autonomy, and how it operated with regard to one's body, emotion and its expression, or individual and family privacy, appeared to reflect conflicting trends within different segments of white British society. A public discourse about children's rights to determine what happened to their feelings and their bodies combined with parental concern not to exert influence on their children's choices. Indeed, there appeared to be an anxiety that *any* influence that was *discernible* risked being (viewed as) *undue* influence, making it more likely that parents would leave essential socialising guidance to peer groups or professionals. For example, these parents appeared to have left guidance about the moral, ethical, and personal consequences of sexual activity to the expertise of school-based sex-education (professional and peer driven), or, triggered by their daughter's tragic and traumatic induction to it, to therapists. As obvious from the two vignettes above neither set of parental decisions assured their child of sufficient information to negotiate the choices and risks that have become a daily part of many children's worlds, nor were they equipped to deal with the far-reaching consequences of experiences that were not reversed by the simple provision of advice on 'sexual health' or easier access to contraception.

Conclusions

It is not surprising that bodies of theory change slowly, lagging behind population movements (both political and geographical) and changes in social structures and values. However, it is possible that certain fields, such as mental health, show a particular resistance to change, attributable perhaps to the fact that its relatively low status as an academic discipline attracts less interest among the best new entrants to medicine and among bodies that fund research. This ambivalence is also apparent in the attitudes of wider society towards the euphemistic distancing of 'mental illness' as 'mental health issues', while claiming to fight the stigma associated with it. While attitudes to professionals, experts and the authority they wield change as fast as the population of 'users' of such expertise, this paper deals with the responsibility that professionals bear to inform public perceptions and expectations. Traditions of expertise that arise within any one culture may not claim universal authority. This is especially important in a field as context-dependent, with as many rapid shifts and contradictions, as child mental health. Equally, no single discipline may claim access to all the 'truths' of how children develop, and which skills will equip them best to survive within the diversity of circumstances they find themselves in. Indeed, the uncertainty in many parts of the world about the survival of children into adulthood, is accompanied by an equal uncertainty about the worlds that successive generations will inhabit. What might a responsible and reflexive professional system contribute to such uncertainty? A robust re-defintion of expertise must lay to rest the obsolete, positivistic expectation of a psychological discipline that pursues scientific 'purity' by excluding the real-life difficulties posed by cultural change. Expertise in the field of child mental health must be based on a tradition of research and theory-building that is responsive to local contexts rather than on inherited authority, or universalising claims based on prestige. It must also embrace inter-disciplinary exchange and promote periodic re-evaluations of the databases on which policy is reliant if it is to remain relevant to local and contemporary circumstances, and responsive to the local needs and risks of children.

"The difficulty is that our judgements of the rationality of each other's discourses about those objects will always be couched within the causal hypotheses embedded in our own discourse. Our representations, albeit of the same objects, are being pulled in different directions by their embeddedness in different systems of signification. When we fail to match their representations to an object whose existence we concede, the traditional anthropological strategies have been either to dismiss their discourse as irrational . . ., or . . ., to assert that the real object is not the one posited by indigenous discourse. . . . I argue that a preferable strategy is to suspend our judgement and allow sufficient cognitive 'space' for conflicting ontologies to exist." (Layton, 1997: 128)

And finally, while the continuing demand for expertise in the 'health' arena is likely to remain, fuelled by its value as a major political counter, the influence of the professions on future opinion and policy is likely to change. It is especially important to be wary of the temptation to make unjustifiable claims for the mental health disciplines, fired by a political climate of endless demand for 'innovation', and to periodically weigh up the validity and impact of our intrusions into the domain of private relationships. In a throwaway line, Archard (1993: 120) warns against an overemphasis on the privacy of the family – *". . ., arguments to the effect that the public can be familialised, that is that all our social relationships can be transformed to resemble a large family are simply naïve."* In defence of such forms of naivete one would wish to cite the impressive variety of bridges which individuals build to make separateness (or isolation from one's family and group) bearable. One might argue that these solutions promote a reciprocity and altruism that bring other benefits in train, and are preferable to an over-reliance on professional relationships for the ordinary losses, hurts and grievances that life necessarily brings. In a climate of ambivalent regard for expertise, it is essential for mental health professionals to revitalise their fields, to abandon traditional islands of authority and enter fully into the richness of inter-disciplinary debate, research and a re-examination of the validity of its constructs.

". . . nothing said yet
now we're speaking
well we're going well
me is asking questions
worker is answering
well something's wrong
I think I got to investigate
. . .
someone is mad now
bla bla bla comment comment comment
hey! that's not right is it
still the same person
we're not getting anywhere
. . ."

(Child, aged 8, at a child protection conference)

References

Archard, D. (1993) *Children: Rights and Childhood.* London: Routledge.

Ariés, P. (1996) *Centuries of Childhood.* London: Pimlico.

Aynsley-Green, A (2003) Practical Implications of the Emerging NSF for Children on 22 Jan 2003
http://www.dh.gov.uk/PolicyAndGuidance/HealthAndSocialCareTopics/ChildrenServices/ChildrenServicesInformation/ChildrenServicesInformation
Article/fs/en?CONTENT_ID=4073061&chk=8LFCtE (downloaded on 26.3.05)

BBC News (2 Sep 2004) French scarf ban comes into force.
http://news.bbc.co.uk/go/pr/fr/-/1/hi/world/europe/3619988.stm

Boyden, J. (1997) Childhood and the policy makers. In A. James and A. Prout (eds) *Constructing and Reconstructing Childhood: Contemporary issues in the Sociological study of childhood.* (2nd ed). London: Falmer Press.

Boynton, P.M., Wood, G.W. and Greenhalgh, T. (2004) Hands-on guide to questionnaire research Reaching beyond the white middle classes. *British Medical Journal,* 328, 1433-1436.

Carsten, J. (2000) *Cultures of Relatedness New Approaches to the Study of Kinship.* Cambridge: Cambridge University Press.

Coote, A. Allen, J. and Woodhead, D, (2004) *Finding Out What Works: Building knowledge about complex, community-based initiatives.* London: Kings Fund Publications.

Das, V. (2003) (ed) *The Oxford India Companion to Sociology and Social Anthropology. Volumes I and II.* New Delhi: OUP.

Dasen, P. R. (2003) Theoretical frameworks in cross-cultural developmental psychology: An attempt at integration. In (ed) T.S. Saraswathi *Cross-Cultural Perspectives in Human Development*. New Delhi: Sage.

Dembour, M. (2001) Following the movement of a pendulum: between universalism and relativism. In: J.K. Cowan, M. Dembour and R.A. Wilson (eds) *Culture and Rights Anthropological Perspectives*. Cambridge University Press.

Donzelot, J. (1997) *The Policing of Families*. Translated from the French by R. Hurley. Baltimore: Johns Hopkins University Press.

Dyer, C. (2004) News: GMC decision on Southall is challenged as "unduly lenient". *British Medical Journal*, October, 329, p 815.

Freud, S. (1973) *2. New Introductory Lectures on Psychoanalysis*. London: Penguin.

Giddens, A. (1991) *Modernity and Self-Identity: Self and society in the late modern age*. Cambridge: Polity Press.

Hall, C. (1996) Histories, empires and the post-colonial moment. In I. Chambers and L. Curti (eds) *The Post-Colonial Question Common Skies Divided Horizons*. London: Routledge.

Hannerz, U. (2002) Notes on the Global Ecumene. In J.X. Inda and R. Rosaldo (eds) *The Anthropology of Globalization A Reader*. Blackwell Publishing

Harris, J. (2005) Emerging Third World powers: China, India and Brazil. *Race & Class*, 46(3), 7-27.

Hill, P. (1993) Recent advances in selected aspects of adolescent development. *Journal of Child Psychology and Psychiatry*, 34 (1), 69-99.

James, A. (1998) Imaging children 'At home', 'In the family' and 'At school': Movement between the spatial and temporal markers of childhood identity in Britain. In N Rapport and A Dawson (eds) *Migrants of Identity Perceptions of Home in a World of Movement*. Oxford: Berg Publishers.

Kagitçibasi, C. (1996) The autonomous-relational self: a new synthesis. *European Psychologist*, 1, 180-186.

Keller, H., Yovsi, R., Borke, J., Kärtner, J., Jensen, H. and Papaligoura, Z. (2004) Developmental consequences of early parenting experiences: Self-recognition and self-regulation in three cultural communities. *Child Development*, 75,6,1745-1760.

Kessel, F.S. and Siegel, A.W. (Eds) (1983) *The Child and Other Cultural Inventions*. New York: Praeger.

Kessen, W. (1983) The child and other cultural inventions. In (Eds) F.S. Kessel, and A.W. Siegel *The Child and Other Cultural Inventions*. New York: Praeger.

Kirmayer, L.J. and Minas, H. (2000) The Future of Cultural Psychiatry: An international perspective. *Canadian Journal of Psychiatry*, 45, 438-446.

Krause, I.B. (1998) *Therapy across Culture*. London: Sage.

Krause, I.B. (in press) Hidden Points of view in cross-cultural psychotherapy and ethnography. *Transcultural Psychiatry*.

Larkin, B. (2002) Indian films and Nigerian lovers: Media and the creation of parallel modernities. In J.X. Inda and R. Rosaldo (eds) *The Anthropology of Globalization A Reader*. Blackwell Publishing

Lau, A. (1984) Transcultural issues in Family Therapy. *Journal of Family Therapy*, 6, 91-112.

Layton, R. (1997) Representing and translating people's place in the landscape of northern Australia. In A. James, J. Hockey and A. Dawson (Eds) *After Writing Culture Epistemology and Praxis in Contemporary Anthropology*. London: Routledge.

Le Vine, R.A., Dixon, S., Le Vine, S., Richman, A., Herbert Leiderman, P., Keefer, C.H. and Brazelton, T.B. (1996) *Child Care and Culture: Lessons from Africa*. Cambridge: Cambridge University Press.

Liljestrom, R. (1983) The Public child, the commercial child and our child. In Kessel, F.S. and Siegel, A.W. (Eds) (1983) *The Child and Other Cultural Inventions*. New York: Praeger.

Maitra, B. (1995) Giving due consideration to families racial and cultural backgrounds. In P Reder and C Lucey (Eds) *Assessment of Parenting: Psychiatric and Psychological Considerations*. London: Routledge.

Maitra, B. (1996) Child abuse: A universal "diagnostic" category ? The implication of culture in definition and assessment. *International Journal of Social Psychiatry*, vol 42, no 4, 287-304.

Maitra, B. (2004a) The cultural relevance of the mental health disciplines. In (Eds) M. Malek and C. Joughin – *Mental Health Services for Minority Ethnic Children and Adolescents*. College Research Unit/Focus Project. London: Royal College of Psychiatrists.

Maitra, B. (2004b) Would cultural matching ensure culturally competent assessments? In (Eds) P. Reder, S. Duncan & C. Lucey - *Studies in the Assessment of Parenting*. London: Routledge.

Maitra, B. (in press) The Many Cultures of Child Protection. In (ed) L. Combrinck-Graham (2nd ed) *Children in Family Context*. NY: Guilford Publications.

McKenzie, K., Patel, V. and Araya, R. (2004) Learning from low income countries: mental health. *British Medical Journal*, 329, 1138-1140.

Nsamenang, A.B. (1992) *Human Development in Cultural Context*. Beverly Hills, CA: Sage.

Offer D., Ostrov E. and Howard K. (1984) *Patterns of Adolescent Self-image*. San Francisco: Jossey-Bass.

Offord D. R., Boyle M. H., Szatinari P., et al (1987) Ontario Child-health study II. Six-month prevalence of disorder and rates of service utilization. *Archives of General Psychiatry*, 44:832-836.

Oxman, A.D., Chalmers, I. And Liberati, A. (2004) A field guide to experts. *British Medical Journal*, 329, 1460-1463.

Prout, A. (2005) *The Future of Childhood*. Oxon: RoutledgeFalmer.

Rogoff, B., Sellers, M.J., Pirrotta, S., Fox, N. and White, S.H. (1975) Age of assignment of roles and responsibilities to children A cross-cultural survey. *Human Development*, 18: 353-369.

Saraswathi, T.S. (2003) (ed) *Cross-Cultural Perspectives in Human Development*. New Delhi: Sage.

Scheper-Hughes, N. (1987) (ed) *Child Survival: Anthropological perspectives on the treatment and maltreatment of children..* Dordrecht, Holland: D. Reidel Publishing Co.

Scheper-Hughes, N. (2003) Culture, scarcity and maternal thinking. In M.G. Spinelli (ed) *Infanticide: Psychosocial and legal perspectives on mothers who kill.* Washington, DC: American Psychiatric Publishing.

Shiva Kumar, A.K. (1998) Economic growth, poverty and child rights: Looking back, looking ahead. In – *A Selection of the Proceedings of a Conference At the Threshold of the Millenium,* Lima, Peru.

Simpson, B. (1997) Representations and the re-presentation of family An analysis of divorce narratives. In A. James, J. Hockey and A. Dawson (Eds) *After Writing Culture: Epistemology and praxis in contemporary anthropology.* London: Routledge.

Strathern, M. (1992) *After Nature English Kinship in the Late Twentieth Century.* Cambridge University Press.

Steinberg, L. (1990) Autonomy, conflict and harmony in the family. In Feldman S.S. and Elliott G.R. (eds) *At the Threshold: The Developing Adolescent.* pp 255-276. Cambridge MA: Harvard University Press.

Super, C.M. and Harkness, S. (1986) The developmental niche: A conceptualization at the interface of child and culture. *International Journal of Behavioural Development,* 9, 545-569.

Timimi, S. (2005) *Naughty Boys: Anti-social behaviour, ADHD and the role of culture.* Basingstoke, Hampshire: Palgrave Macmillan.

Tristan, F. (2005) Opinion, *BMA News* (12 February) p 10.

Tyrer, P. (2005) Combating editorial racism in psychiatric publications. *British Journal of Psychiatry,* 186, 1-3.

Yamada, H. (2004) Japanese mothers' views of young children's areas of personal discretion. *Child Development,* 75, 1, p 164-179.

Whiting, B.B. and Whiting, J.W.M. (1975) *Children of Six Cultures: A psycho-cultural analysis.* Cambridge, MA: Harvard University Press.

4

Childhood: An Indian Perspective

Rajeev Banhatti · Kedar Dwivedi · Begum Maitra

"I do not want my house to be walled in on all sides, and my windows to be closed. Instead, I want the cultures of all lands to be blown about my house as freely as possible. But I refuse to be blown off my feet by any."

Mahatma Gandhi

Introduction

This chapter, by three child psychiatrists of Indian origin practising in Britain, is a very brief account of Indian childhoods. It will explore the ways in which ideas about children are part of the fabric of cultural beliefs about other aspects of Indian life. They encompass a wide variety of personal and transpersonal concerns within any society, but reflect and respond to particular physical, social, and historical contexts. This is not an attempt to encompass the history, politics, and religion, not to mention psychology, of a region so large and varied in a single chapter. We aim only to pick out a small number of themes relevant to children, and to illustrate how these may be traced back to the shared past of the people in the Indian subcontinent. From this past arose ideas about what made a good life, exemplary tales of children and their relationships, mythologies, and religious traditions that, filtered through memory and re-constructions, create the particular repertoire of contemporary beliefs and practices that make for an 'Indian' childhood. By virtue of its brevity this chapter reflects a personal selection from the many ways in which Indian history and culture may be described. The authors make no claims to greater 'authenticity' in this account, or to 'accuracy' of representation. In defence of this apparently lamentable disregard for scientific rigour we argue that since all cultures change with re-telling, cultural transmission to successive generations (the inheritors of their parents versions of culture) cannot be other than idiosyncratic. Furthermore, when a group is faced with sudden change or its autonomy appears under threat, as in migrant groups or during 'ethnic' wars, it is both likely to be opportunistic in how it selects from its cultural rules, and to defend this culture as authentic tradition. We are also hoping to answer more fully some questions we have been asked about our culture, but not had the presence of mind or the skill to hold our interlocutor's attention as we drew a long breath to explain! Questions that start "*Why* do Indians (do this or that)[1]. . .?" cannot have short answers. Cultural practices, even those most recently invented or borrowed, rarely have short histories. In fact, their basis in cross-cutting systems of belief that are often only partly conscious make attempts to 'explain' them complex and long-winded. This chapter touches on the areas relevant to understanding how cultures work, such as history, ancient and modern, religion and myth, ethnoscience and healing, and the interested reader may wish to explore these further.

This chapter focuses on only one among the many South Asian cultures, and from among the numerous other world cultures that may be relevant to British clinicians. However, it does so without apology. Few papers that deal with clinical issues simultaneously address background cultural matters at any length, and lists of ethnic groups, languages, religious and dietary customs are of little help in understanding the fine detail of emotional lives and relationships. We hope that this chapter will add to the body of ethnographic and cross-cultural literature about childhoods around the world. Further, while we focus on India, it is necessary to remember that the contemporary nations of Pakistan, Bangladesh and India were separated just over half a century ago, but are united by a long and shared cultural history. These antecedents shape and colour the lives of the possibly half billion children in India alone, and inevitably influence the cultural environments of children in the other two countries, as well as those of innumerable children of the South Asian diaspora around the world.

Hinduism, as a collection of beliefs and practices, is the oldest strand of continuity within the sub-continent. Demographically dominant[2] among the Indic religions (that include Buddhism, Jainism and Sikhism), Hinduism wields a hegemonic influence over the great diversity of cultures within contemporary India (Madan, 2003), and gives a particular colouring also to the religions that originated outside India (namely, Christianity, Islam, Judaism, Zoroastrianism and the Bahai faith). While a focus on Hinduism may appear odd, even unwarranted, in a book on psychological and health perspectives on children, Madan (*ibid*, p 776) writes of the place of religion in Indian cultural life –

'. . . *religion in India is not a discrete element of everyday life that stands wholly apart from the economic or political concerns of the people. . . . The point is not that the religious domain is not distinguished from the secular, but rather that the secular is regarded as being encompassed by the religious, even when the former is apparently inimical to the latter. The*

---

[1] The disappointing thing about such questions is the fact that the questioner is rarely sufficiently informed to ask the really interesting questions, or to be interested in the response! There is little real pleasure to be had from rhetorical questions such as "Do you believe in arranged marriages?"

[2] Four of five Indians are Hindu.

relationship is hierarchical. In other words, religion in the Indian cultural setting traditionally permeates virtually all aspects of life, not through mechanical diffusion, but in an integrated, holistic perspective . . .'.

History, Society and Religion

Debates rage over historical accounts of a nation, the authenticity and dating of ancient sources, hierarchical relationships and vested interests. As Saumarez-Smith (2003, p 100) points out, there are distinct traditions of historiography – the European, Sanskritic and Islamic traditions among others – and that each historical version impacts on subsequent events[3] – "*The writing of history goes into the making of nations and cannot suddenly be unwritten.*" The writing of ancient histories of countries such as India might suffer particularly from the dearth of textual sources, and may also be open to the vagaries of intellectual fashions. Thapar (1966) comments on the rise and fall of European interest in Indian culture and religion, noting that both colonial British disdain and German romanticism wrought considerable havoc on Indians' perceptions of themselves. The dichotomy created in the nineteenth century between the 'spirituality' of Indian values and the 'materialism' of the West had little interest in placing this spirituality within the context of Indian society. Further, early European enquiries into Indian culture relied on Brahmin priests as informants and on Sanskrit sources, neglecting the rich cultures of the Indian south. Their accounts of the history of the region were mainly concerned with the rise and fall of empires and dynasties, and preoccupied with comparisons with the classical (Greek) tradition of Europe. When taken over by Indian historians of the late nineteenth and twentieth centuries, keen to promote nationalist aspirations, these accounts were intent on showing the glory of ancient India before the arrival of the colonisers.

The following brief historical account of the civilisations in the Indian sub-continent is supported by archaeological evidence. The earliest traces of human activity in the region go back to the Second Inter-Glacial period (400,000 and 200,000 B.C). The slow evolution of human settlements in the North-Western regions resulted in the spectacular Indus Valley Civilization (or the Harappa Culture) around 2500 B.C. This essentially urban culture (in Punjab and Sind of modern-day Pakistan, and the Rajasathan and Kathiawar regions in India) was focussed mainly in the cities of Mohenjo-Daro and Harappa, conducting a flourishing trade with the Persian Gulf and Mesopotamia. The arrival in this region of Indo-Aryans from Iran in about 1500 B.C.

---

[3] A particularly interesting critique of elitist historiography grew in the 1980s with the Subaltern Studies movement (Guha, 1982), that proposed a change of perspective from the bird's eye view to worm's eye-view, from official to subaltern, It helped to promote significant research and writing on tribal and peasant histories.

brought in new cultural elements that contributed to the evolution of the distinctive Vedic culture in the north; other cultures developed in the central regions of the Deccan and the valley of the Ganga (Ganges), and in southern India. Information about this period is also based on stone engravings of Buddhist teachings and a large body of Sanskrit scriptures and literature that is available only through the tradition of oral transmission among Hindu (Brahmin) priests. (See Dwivedi and Prasad, 2000 for further details).

Ideas from the Vedic period had a seminal influence over how society[4], and childhood, were conceptualised. The impact of these ancient sources is evident in the character of contemporary beliefs about children in India, and marks their radically different character from the evolution of Western ideas about the nature of childhood. Indian concerns about children, and the purpose of childhood, were formed by ideas about the purpose of life on earth, and the goals of child-rearing were to foster those abilities needed in the performance of certain duties, and for the maintenance of particular values (*samskaras*). More will be said about this later, after a brief account of the impact of major influences from outside the subcontinent.

Mediaeval India saw a period of peace and affluence for about a millennium, with the rise of the arts and crafts, and advances in music and literature. This golden age of Indian culture is evident in the famous temples and sculptures that still stand from this period, and in travelogues by Chinese scholars like Miuen Tsiang. Invasions from the North by Afghans and Turks brought new influences into northern India, including Islamic religion and culture. The destruction and looting of temples motivated by their enormous wealth, was to remain in the Hindu mind, colouring perceptions of Muslim rulers (Thapar, 1966, p 233). Despite the episodic coercion and violence of kings, the spread of Islam was slow, depending initially on Hindu converts[5]. Tradition states that Christianity arrived in India with Saint Thomas in the first century, and grew with the arrival of Jesuit missionaries in the sixteenth century. Present day Christians of all denominations in India have retained many of their pre-conversion beliefs, attitudes and ceremonies, incorporating them into Christianity. Contrary to the assumptions about the exclusive nature of religious faith there is considerable evidence of religious pluralism in India, both in ancient and modern times. As Madan asserts "*The common people of India acknowledge religious difference as the experienced reality: they do not consider it good or bad.*" (2003, p 798).

---

[4] For example, developing the concept of divine kingship, an administrative system and the patriarchal family as the unit of society; contributing to the evolution of a caste system based on race, social origins and occupation, and not originally hereditary.

[5] Madan (2003) notes that despite 800 years of Muslim rule, no more than a quarter of the population were Muslim when the Partition of India and Pakistan took effect in 1947.

Colonisation and its impact

Unlike the Mughal rulers of India, very few British settled in India, the main purpose of colonisation being economic, and intended to strengthen the British economy, industry and political power. However, colonial rule was accompanied by propaganda that presented it as beneficial for the advancement of the native population, a benefit that was to be achieved by emulating the British way of life as much as possible. Nandy (1999) hypothesised that in the context of British colonialism in India, progress was conceptualised as a reformation of the 'childlike' Indian (innocent, ignorant but willing to learn, loyal and grateful) by 'Westernisation', modernization or Christianisation. The 'childish' Indian (ignorant but unwilling to learn, ungrateful, sinful, savage, disloyal and incorrigible), on the other hand, was to be moulded by repression, brute force and a tough rule of law and administration. These measures would, it was hoped, make coloniser and colonised partners in realising a world that was culturally and politically homogeneous. This colonization of Indian minds has been very damaging in the long term. The process of 'decolonization' (Nederveen Pieterse and Parekh, 1995) has required individual and collective struggles to establish what is Indian, and to distinguish it from reactions to the West, whether positive or negative. '*The pressure to be the obverse of the West distorts the traditional priorities in the Indian's total view of man and universe and destroys his culture's unique gestalt. It in fact binds him even more irrevocably to the West*' (Nandy, 1999, p 8).

Many middle and lower ranks of administrators were sent to outposts of the British Empire around the world, and their descendents, along with the numbers transported as indentured labour[6], form the earliest cohorts of the Indian diaspora abroad. Freedom was already a lost and cherished ideal for the Indian society and it was rediscovered during the 18th and 19th century as the Indian nationalist movement took root. When British rule came to an end in 1947 two countries were born, India and Pakistan. Pakistan was a Muslim country and India was a parliamentary democracy committed to secularism. Ambedkar, a Buddhist, was one of the main architects of this secular constitution, formalised in 1950, which outlawed negative discrimination on the basis of caste and religion and urged affirmative action to help those traditionally disadvantaged.

Indian democracy has evolved through many upheavals since independence. The early post independence era was marked by optimism, socialism and

---

[6] Under an 'indentured' or contract labour of forced labour that resembled enslavement, Indians, began to replace enslaved Africans on plantations across the British empire, in Fiji, Natal, Burma, Ceylon, Malaya, British Guiana, Jamaica and Trinidad in the mid-19th century.

cautious non-alignment through the cold war era. The mid 1990s saw a greater liberalising of Indian economic policies, resulting in a boom in computing and information technology, and rapid change in urban Indian society. The greater opportunities and affluence ushered in by this period has had a particular impact on Indian adolescents and young adults who were able to compete for employment and business opportunities abroad.

Cultural Ideologies and Practices

Aryan influence on the culture of the indigenous people of north western India resulted in the development of Vedic religion. Vedic ideas and practices were then theorised and elaborated during the Upanishadic (or Vedantic) period. Heterodox schools, such as Charwaks, Jainism and Buddhism emerged as challenges to Vedic authority.

Both Hinduism and Buddhism contain the concept of human existence as an endless cycle of birth and rebirth through a variety of possible forms (including gods, demons, animals, etc.) until the ultimate aim is achieved, that of liberation of the self/soul (*atman*) from this cycle. In Hinduism this liberation is known as *moksha*, in Buddhism it is *nirvana* (Enlightenment). Vedic religion remains visible in its successor, modern Hinduism. Thapar (1966) traces some of the familiar notions of contemporary Hinduism from these ancient sources – *dharma* (the natural law), the doctrine of *karma* (or the consequences of *action* in past lives), and the four *ashramas* ('refuges', or stages of life). In Hinduism, the self (*atman)* was considered timeless and formless, manifesting itself in the physical body, which is considered no more than its outer garment, due to the nature of past actions. The ultimate goal of *moksha* was achievable through the practice of *dharma* and the accumulation of merit through right action. The routes to self-realisation in Hinduism are numerous and vary with the nature and abilities of the individual – and include meditation, devotion (*bhakti*) to man or to God, yoga, and asceticism.

The cluster of Indian ideas around the notions of *karma* and reincarnation are of particular relevance to considerations of motivation, causal relationships and responsibility. Cantile (2003) notes that there is a tendency in the Indian explanation of day-to-day events to blur the distinction between what a man is and what happens to him. She gives the example of why the body of a murdered man is denied funeral rites, noting in a manner that is likely to seem impossibly elliptical to the Western reader, that

"... *he was such a man that this happened to him. . . . Speaking mythologically, we can say, first, that a man prefigures the events of his life which he attracts to himself; second, that through these events, seen in reverse, as it were, he is shown to us – and possibly to himself – as being what he is; and third, that the plot of his life unfolds in the space of these two perspectives."* (Cantile, 2003, p 830).

Yet other aspects of the Indian orientation to the material world may be seen as arising from the principles discussed above. Thus, the transient and essentially illusory nature of the material world suggests that the ideal attitude towards worldly success may be to disregard it, and to denigrate competitiveness as *himsa* (a concept that combines aggressiveness with greed/envy). While these are admittedly ideals, and as in any other culture are neither valued equally by all, nor adhered to uniformly, they form the background of expectations upon which Indians are likely to experience satisfaction, and pride/shame in themselves, their families and their achievements. Equally, these attitudes allow an easier acceptance, and accommodation to, misfortune, ill health and imperfections in others. This insistence on tolerance and fortitude frequently appears to Western viewers as fatalism, passivity, or even as a response of 'learned helplessness' to the chronic poverty within the region. On the contrary, it must be understood as part of the Indian emphasis on humility, and the vision of man as one link in a cycle that connects him to all other sentient beings. The Western notion of man as the pinnacle of all creation (and made in the image of the divine) lends to this culture vastly different ideas of man's rightful role in conquest, and in mastery over animals and all of nature.

In Buddhism the Self is considered to be a product of illusory processes that arise as a consequence of the enormous speed of mental activity. The practice of meditation helps to develop concentration (mindfulness) and the capacity to penetrate these illusory processes. This process gradually leads to enlightenment, but may take many lifetimes. In order to continue working for enlightenment, it is necessary that future births occur in a suitable plane of existence. By adhering to the rules of virtuous and moral living, which also form the foundation for practicing meditation, one may ensure (through the laws of *karma* in both Hinduism and Buddhism) that rebirth will occur in a higher plane of existence (Dwivedi, 1990).

Ethnopsychology – Emotion, thought and personality

The cross-cultural study of emotions show how these are socially constructed. Culture influences the way emotions are understood, processed, and expressed, and in its function of allocating meaning to experience. It also helps determine what may be considered 'traumatic', and the severity of trauma (Dwivedi, 2000, Dwivedi and Varma 1997, Lokare, 1997, Maitra, 1995 and 2004).

Western attempts to study emotion have mainly focussed on its physiological bases and functions, and have tended to dismiss the emotions as 'irrational'. On the other hand, the social significance of emotion in India is accorded a centrality though the theory of '*Rasa*'. Established several millennia ago as evidenced by Bharat's *Natyashastra* of 200 BC (de Bary et al 1958, Dwivedi and Gardner 1997), this system of beliefs cultivates and refines the experience and expression of emotions through art, literature, stories and drama.

> '*The experience of the rasa is a glimpse of and, more important, an experience of the divine bliss inherent in all humans*' (Lynch 1990, p 18).
> and
> '*Contrary to Western devaluation of emotion in the face of reason, India finds emotions, like food, necessary for a reasonable life, and, like taste, cultivable for the fullest understanding of life's meaning and purpose. . . . in much of India there is no real distinction between mind and body, cognition and emotion, and asceticism and eroticism.*' (Lynch, *ibid.*, p 23)

Indeed, emotion is considered to link the personal sphere to the material and spiritual realms, and there is a considerable emphasis on emotion regulation in the Indian culture (Dwivedi, 2002, 2004, Roland 1980). In Buddhism, 'mindfulness' of the emotions can be a means of practicing meditation, and a path to the achievement of *nirvana* or enlightenment.

These traditions of thought, while religious (and Hindu) in origin, pervade everyday cultural exchanges – through art, music, myth, narrative, folk theatre, dance – and it would be unusual for someone growing up in India not to be influenced by these in one way or another. It is perhaps to this pervasiveness of the symbolic, conceptual and affective elements of Hindu religious mythology that Cantile (2003, p 827) refers when she writes ". . ., *India offers to the mythologist a field for the study of living myths which has not ceased to be cultivated from ancient times to the present.*" With telling examples that would be hard to present briefly here[7], Cantile discusses the 'Indian' way of thinking within a 'myth-history continuum' that cancels and confuses both terms. However, she adds that it " . . . *has a kind of self-awareness which recognizes the metaphors of its own thinking.*" (p 631). According to Kakar (1997), the emphasis in Indian culture is on being more inward focussed (mindful), with thought being marked more by primary process and synthesis rather than analysis. Experience and emotion, and submersion in these, may be more appealing to the Indian mind than the outward looking, secondary process thinking allegedly characteristic of Western modes, and its valuing of rationality, analysis, categorisation and classification.

Indian researchers (Kapur et al, 1995) have developed the Developmental

---

[7] For example, she refers to the simultaneous mythical and modern significance of Ayodhya in India which, as the mythical birthplace of the Hindu god Ram, became the site of real-life conflict. The political motivations undoubtedly served by such conflict would be ineffectual without the emotive power of the myth.

Psychopathology Check List (DPCL) that operationalises this theory of temperament, doing so on the same lines as the classic New York Longitudinal Study by Thomas and Chess (1977), and undertaken studies of its reliability. In a study (Kapur et al, 1997) of 50 Indian pre-school children they found that 26 had Satvik temperaments (good natured and well adjusted), 14 Rajasik (highly-strung/active), and 5 had Tamasik (torpid/dull) temperaments. (The remaining 5 did not have a predominant predisposition.) It is likely that this system will be of enormous clinical significance due to the 'better fit' with parental and societal expectations in India.

India is the birthplace of two classical medical systems – *Ayurveda* ('science of life') and *Siddha*, and according to Kakar (1982, p 220) *Ayurveda* is the *"principal repository of the Indian cultural image of the body"*. It offers a systematic understanding of the effects of differing foods, hygienic practices, occupational exposures, seasonal and geographic influences, cosmological forces, spiritual presences, and the moral consequences of social actions in the present and previous lives. *Ayurveda*'s theory of *triguna*[8] (three *guna* loosely translated as dispositions) recognises three intrinsic properties of the mind and matter with a common origin. These are – *satvik* (pure and altruistic, a very positive quality); *rajasik* (active and positive, but not pure); *tamasik* – (inactive, lazy or obstructive, a negative quality). Rather like temperament these are intrinsic to the child, the baby possessing these *guna* in different proportions. These may be discerned during pregnancy, when *satvik* qualities may be increased by prescribing corrective diet and activities to the mother. This process may be continued after birth as diet, massage and medicinal treatments aimed at the child.

Child Development and Parental Duties

Concepts of childhood and attitudes towards children change, being rooted in their own times and cultures. In early 17th century Europe children were considered innately evil, born with 'original sin 'due to the puritan dogma (Aries, 1962), and it was the duty of adults to purge them of this by persuasion, or by measures that were often harsh and punitive. The British philosopher

---

[8] This Triguna theory is also linked to Sankhya philosophy, which considered the three gunas as modes of being, or tendencies of existence, that are like three strands which are twisted together making a rope. That rope is *Prakriti*, the female half of cosmic substance in a dualistic theory of the universe. When *Prakriti* is in its perfectly balanced state the universe is non-manifest. On contact with *Purusha*, the masculine half of the cosmic substance the balance is disturbed setting a chain reaction, which leads to manifest matter and mind which is formed of an imperfect combination of the gunas.

Locke (1632-1704) was responsible in part for a radical shift in the collective view of the child as a 'blank slate', and a product of the environment it developed in. Rousseau, and 18th century European romanticism, further developed the image of children as born innocent, pure and naturally good.

Indian beliefs about children present them as gifts of the divine life force, and as complex entities even at birth. Present day concepts of the child and its development, as well as of the duties of parents and how child care may best be provided, may be identified within ancient tradition. While there is some variation of practice according to region and class/caste membership, Kakar (1997) describes the five stages of childhood most widely known, noting also the rites of transition and the central relationship patterns in each stage.

Childhood period	Stage	Central mode of relationship	Rite marking the transition into following stage
i. *Garbha*	1. Foetus	Symbiotic	*Jatakarma*
ii. *Ksheerda*	2. Early infancy (0-1 month)	Dyadic intimacy	*Namakarana*
	3. Middle infancy (1-3/4 months)	Dyad in family	*Nishkramana*
	4. Late infancy (3/4-6/9 months)	Dyad in world	*Anna prasana*
iii. *Ksheerannada*	5. Early childhood (6/9 months-2/3 yrs)	Dyadic dissolution (psychological birth)	*Chudakarana*
iv. *Bala*	6. Middle childhood (2/3-5/7 years)	Familial	*Vidyarambha*
v. *Kumara*	7. Late childhood (5/7-8/12 years)	Familial dissolution (social birth)	*Upanayana*

Stages of Childhood: The Hindu Scheme of Social development (Kakar, 1997, p 208)

The ideological model of *ashramas*, life stages, complements this system, continuing from childhood to the stages of later life. The emphasis on appropriate relationships, tasks and duties suggests that the goals of development centralise collective social aims through much of life. The more individualistic goals (spiritual rather than material) appear in old age.

- *balakashram* – (infancy to school age; *balak* young child). A period of self-indulgence and indulgence by adults, in which parents, but more often grandparents and elders narrate stories from mythology, folk tales and local legend, to entertain but also to inspire and induct children into cultural modes of feeling and thinking.

- *brahmacharyashram* (phase of self-denial and celibacy from school age to adolescence; *brahmacharya* celibacy). The *gurukul* (*guru* teacher, *kul* home) tradition of ancient India required children to live and study in the forest-based schools of teachers for the entire period, ensuring their concentration on acquiring knowledge and skills. Some contemporary Indian boarding schools adopt a modified approach with a suitably adapted curriculum to fit current needs.

- *grihasthashrama* (family life; *grihastha* householder) The phase of marriage and family life extending up to the completion of one's duties to one's children (namely, their reaching maturity as marked by their marriages).

- *vanaprasthashrama* (*vanaprastha* forest dweller). Gradual renunciation of mundane concerns in middle to old age

- *sanyasa* (*sanyas* renouncer) An optional phase entered into by a small minority, which required total renunciation of all material possessions and relationships, with the development of non-attachment as its goal.

Samskaras and socialisation

Hindu tradition specifies rites of passage (*samskara*) for the individual, which mark an incremental process of attaining adult community identity as the individual journeys through the life course. While many of these are only for male children, some *samskaras* are only for girls, and women have prescribed roles in the ceremonies. The naming ceremony for both boys and girls is performed by the parents and grandparents, under the guidance of a priest versed in Sanskrit prayers. It is an occasion for singing and feasting with the community. *Upanayana,* the sacred thread ceremony, is conducted at any time between the eighth and twelfth year, and marks the child's 'second (social) birth' into the wider community. It symbolises a boy's transition from that of 'innocent' child to one who is more socially accountable for his actions, and also marks a breaking away from the maternal bond. While few families may practice the most traditional *upanayana* rituals it is still considered an essential rite by most Hindu Indians.

The word *samskara* has also come to mean 'good manners' or acceptable, desirable behaviours. In today's increasingly nuclearised urban families, and among Indians living outside India, there is a lack of family elders who are knowledgeable about ritual, or hold much authority within the family. This has led to the setting up of *Samskara* 'lessons' (resembling scouts or girl guides groups) for children. Run by enthusiastic volunteers these are useful in shaping children's core cultural values, and conveying a sense of cultural self or identity.

Much of the ancient Indian literature is heavily biased in favour of boys, sons and males, the most notable of these texts being the *Manu Smriti*, believed to have been composed between 200 BC and AD 300. While a woman is venerated everywhere as mother, she must as wife, remain subordinate to her husband and male kin. However, this places on men the obligation to protect kinswomen, and on the husband the overriding duty to provide for his family. The ideology of the 'Indian joint family'[9] expected the relations of husband and wife, and parent and child, to be subordinated to the larger collective identity.

It must be noted that there is much regional variation[10] in the degrees of son preference and acceptable levels of female autonomy, as measured by literacy rates, work participation rates, women's inheritance rights, and freedom of divorce and remarriage (Uberoi, 2003). A great deal of ethnographic material is available on Hindu traditions and life-cycle rituals (especially on female puberty, marriage and childbirth), and historical and feminist reassessments of the social reforms of the colonial period (notably, the abolition of *sati*[11] and female infanticide, the raising of the legal age of marriage and the regulation of female sexuality within Sanskritic and Victorian standards of propriety) While relatively little is known of how contemporary urban milieus affect the sexual and reproductive lives of girls and women many writers have commented on the influence of 'kinship ideologies' and culturally embedded ideas of sexuality and procreation on Indian law and administrative structures.

Much less emphasis has been given on the less public, but no less strong, theme of affection and co-operation between male and female kin. A number of contemporary festivals and ceremonies, such as '*Bhaidweej*' and '*Raksha-bandhan*'[12] (*raksha* protection, *bandhan* bond, tie), honour and celebrate the

---

[9] The Hindu joint family is constituted by a group of persons related in the male line and subject to the absolute power of the seniormost member. It has been widely held up as the 'traditional' form of family in India, and as a living example of the earliest or 'ancient' form of the human family, discernible in the legal system of ancient Rome. Its claim as a unifying civilizational ideal excludes other forms of Indian kinship – the Dravidian systems of Southern India, and those of tribal societies and non-Hindu groups.

[10] In general the northern regions are more masculinist on most measures, and the south much less so, with the eastern regions showing mixed characteristics.

[11] This refers to the ritual immolation of a woman on the funeral pyre of her deceased spouse.

[12] The ceremony consists of a symbolic exchange between brothers and sisters that lays reciprocal obligations on both. Thus a *rakhi*, a decorative wrist band tied by a sister onto a brother's wrist, or a dot of sandalwood paste on the brother's forehead, marks the duties of each to honour and protect the other according to rules of their society.

bonds between brothers and sisters. Children are taught to participate in these rituals from early childhood under parental guidance, and acquire an appreciation of the life-long obligations between them.

Legend tells of how the custom of tying rakhis transcended religious boundaries and during Mughal times helped bind Rajput (Hindu) royalty and the Mughal (Muslim) rulers of Delhi together. It is said that when Bahadur Shah of Gujarat attacked Rani Karnavati of Chittor, she sent a rakhi to the Mughal emperor, Humayun, and requested his help. Bound by the power of the symbol Humayun tried to come to her aid, but he was too late. When he arrived Chittor had already fallen and the Queen had immolated herself according to the Rajput custom, rather than surrender to her enemies.

A facet of Indian (or South Asian) parenting attitudes, towards young children in particular, that has been noted by several writers (Kakar. 1997; Maitra, 1995; Maitra and Miller, 2002) and appears repeatedly in myth and legend is the almost unconditional indulgence accorded by adults (or seen as desirable) towards the unsocialized demands of children below the age of 'understanding'[13]. Kakar (1997, p 103) notes that –

"The main emphasis in the early years of Indian childhood is avoidance of frustration and the enhancement of the pleasurable mutuality of mother and infant, not encouragement of the child's individuation and autonomy."

It would wise to be cautious of an analysis of cultural difference that relies too much on convenient and attractive, but essentially limited, dichotomous categories – such as collectivism/individualism (Hofstede, 1991), or independent/interdependent (Markus and Kitayama, 1991). A study (Joshi and MacLean, 1997) of maternal expectations among Indian, Japanese and English middle class urban mothers, with regard to their children's development in a number of domains (such as education/self-care, compliance, peer interaction, communication, emotional control and environmental independence) illustrates significant similarities. Dissimilarities reflected not only cultural difference but also the fluidity of environmental factors. In general, Indian mothers were found to have a more relaxed attitude about the ages at which they expected their children to develop skills, an observation that has also been reported by other writers (Kakar, 1997; Roland, 1980).

---

[13] See Rogoff et al (1975) for similar patterns across many cultures that assign social responsibility to children between the ages of 5-7 years.

The use of myths and folk tales

Many cultures, including that of India, use mythological tales, legends and folk stories as an important means of communicating cultural expectations, providing models of socialisation and solutions to common difficulties that arise in child development and in parental care. Stories and narratives can be therapeutic processes and can have an extremely powerful and transformational influence (Dwivedi, 1997). The two folk stories that follow are well known to Indians, and the fact that no distinctions are made based on the supposed religious 'affiliations' of the characters, point to pan-Indian nature of these images and ideals. The first involves the Mughal (Muslim) Emperor Akbar while the second, about the Hindu god *Hanuman*, forms part of a genre of myths about the childhoods of Hindu gods most prominently figuring the god *Krishna)*. These stories are repeated through life, to entertain children, at religious celebrations, and to illustrate a point in everyday conversations, and reinforce the ideal of parental tolerance towards childish demands. As the stories show, this is often positioned against the competing need to teach children to respect their elders.

Emperor Akbar's punishment to his grandson

> *The Mughal Emperor Akbar liked to present his courtiers with riddles, and had long tried to outwit Birbal, his most wily minister (incidentally, a Hindu). One morning as he was getting ready to go to the court, his little grandson said to him, 'Grandpa, there is something black in your moustache; let me take it out'. When Akbar bent down the child pulled a hair out from his moustache, laughing gleefully at having made his grandfather look foolish. The emperor admonished the child, but smiled secretly to himself. On reaching the court, Emperor Akbar announced angrily that someone had had the insolence to pull a hair from his moustache. 'How', he thundered, 'should the miscreant be punished?'*
>
> *The alarmed courtiers vied to suggest increasingly severe punishments, including sentence of death, but Birbal did not answer and seemed immersed in deep thought. Hoping to have finally outwitted Birbal, Akbar demanded a reply. He was astounded when Birbal bowed, saying 'Jahapanah! (Your Highness) the correct punishment would be a resounding kiss on the cheeks!' The courtiers quivered in fear, thinking that Birbal had finally lost his mind. However, Akbar realised that his minister had again guessed the true circumstances. Asked to explain, Birbal replied: 'Only a child would dare indulging in such a risky prank, and this child could only be your grandson, whom you adore and see every day. Had it been an adult he would surely have been punished immediately.'*

The exploits of Hanuman

Hanuman was born of Vayu, the God of the Wind, and a goddess (Anjana) cursed by a holy man for her rudeness to live as a monkey on earth. The baby monkey's charms made his mother, Anjana, love him dearly; his father gave him the gifts of strength, speed, and the ability to fly.
Hanuman was restless like the wind, but despite his mischievousness he was beloved of all in the monkey world. One day, on seeing the beauty of the sun in the sky the child wanted it for a toy. Surya, the sun god, fled with Hanuman in hot pursuit. Disturbed by the uproar, Indra, king of the gods, hurled a thunderbolt at the flying Hanuman. Vayu found his son in a pitiful state and he howled in fury, causing fierce storms all over the earth. And when he sat on a mountain top, brooding with his lifeless baby in his arms, the world and all creatures suffocated as every day there was less and less air to breathe. The gods appealed to Brahma, the Creator of all life and greater than the king of gods, Indra. Brahma and Indra beseeched Vayu to calm himself, and Indra admitted that he had wrongly succumbed to anger and punishing a mere child too severely. Brahma took Hanuman on his lap and patted him back to life. Mollified, Vayu asked his son to apologise to the gods, and Hanuman complied, as every well brought up child would. He learned also from that day to be calmer, and not take risks unthinkingly.

Some of the ideologies behind parenting patterns in the Indian culture have already been described elsewhere (Dwivedi, 2002) and include attempts to help transcend narcissism and work towards freedom from 'self' with the cultivation of dependability and interdependence (versus independence), extended (versus nuclear) family life, indirect (versus direct and clear) communication.

Contemporary realities and the impact on child mental health

Indian beliefs about the nature of childhood have undergone major changes with the increased global exchange of ideas triggered by economic liberalisation in the mid 1990s. With the widespread impact of computer and information technology (specifically with access to the internet and western cable TV channels) urban Indians are increasingly assimilated into the global homogenised culture dominated by Western values. Parental expectations of their children, the supports available to them from extended family systems, and the boundaries between the family and the outer world are also undergoing change. Kumar (1993) notes that the traditional continuity between the worlds of the Indian child and adult has been disrupted by a number of factors – attendance at school, the demands of parental work schedules, the consumerism (more for the urban middle classes) ushered in by the era of post-liberalisation that has separated children and adolescents, primarily as different segments of the consumer market.

However, as an experienced *Ayurvedic* physician wrote recently –

> *'The child rearing practices and the childcare techniques have been practised over Indian subcontinents for thousands of years from generations to generations with minor changes in different regions and culture. However, no notable bad effects are observed. This has more importance in the light of behavioural disturbances found in children from the so-called developed countries'* (Bhagwat, 2002, p iv).

Yet, it would be unwise to be complacent about the impact of complex environmental and socio-economic realities such as, high rates of maternal and infant mortality among the poor, and the high prevalence of female infanticide in some parts of the country. Other considerations that are commonly cited by Western commentators as harmful to children but are more open to debate, include concerns about parental priorities that do not value formal education, the widespread fact of child labour, early marriage, and the varied forms of 'victimisation' of girls.

One marker of the success or failure of a group to provide 'good enough' contexts for the developmental needs of children might be found in the patterns of emotional disorder in children. *Table 1* summarises the current picture of child mental health concerns in the Indian context. Despite the lack of accurate epidemiological data what is immediately obvious when compared with British data, are the differences in environmental contexts, stressors and patterns of distress

Table 1

	INDIA	UK
Population	1000 million	56.7 million
% of children	40%	20%
Prevalence of psychiatric disorders	8% (Malhotra, 1995) to 30% (Deivasigamani, 1990)	8% (Meltzer et al, 2000)
Common presentations	Pseudoseizures, Dissociative states and Conversion Disorders (e.g. aphonia, paraparesis, sensory loss) ADHD (more recently) OCD	ADHD, Asperger's Syndrome Conduct Disorders Emotional Disorders OCD

	INDIA	UK
Common presentations cont/d...	Psychoses, often organic infective aetiology and delirium. Psychogenic pain, panic attacks	Psychoses, often co-morbid with substance use. Chronic fatigue Syndrome
Common underlying stresses	Poverty, school examinations and performance pressures, physical abuse	Peer related e.g. bullying, sexual abuse, parental separation
Suicide	No reliable data available, rare.	Rare
Attempted suicide and self injury (DSH)	Methods – ingestion of insecticides, self immolation, hanging, wrist cutting. Non-suicidal superficial self harm by cutting or burning – rare	Paracetamol poisoning, hanging. Non-suicidal, self cutting, burning – increasing incidence and common.
Eating Disorders	Very rare and only in the rich westernised section of society before mid-90's. Now, increasing incidence of mild forms. Anorexia and Bulimia remain rare.	Increasing incidence, earlier age of onset. Still seen in girls mainly but increasing incidence in boys.
Western style Treatment Facilities	Only in the larger cities. Elsewhere, practitioners may be unqualified or semi-qualified. Almost no in-patient facilities for children.	Relatively well organised and increasing priority and resources in government policies.

Interestingly, there is some evidence that children of the Indian diaspora show lower prevalence of mental disorder when compared to children from other ethnic minorities, and in Britain, also when compared with the indigenous majority (Banhatti and Bhate, 2002). While it would be too simplistic to attribute this difference to culture alone, it raises the possibility that some aspects of Indian culture may contribute to the greater resilience of these children. And if this were true it would be important to determine which elements of cultural practice in parenting were likely to be significant and how might these be promoted?

Hackett et al (1993) compared parental ideas about normal and deviant child behaviour in Gujarati and English communities in the UK. They found more exacting notions of normality in the Gujarati community, and that these were linked to a lower rate of disturbance in Gujarati children! This effect may well be mediated indirectly through the greater stability of Gujarati families, both providing greater support to children and demanding a higher level of performance on social tasks. It is hoped that this rich arena for further research into cultural resilience will balance the tendency to treat culture in a tokenistic fashion, or to cite it only in explanation of dysfunction[14]. The very least that we might do when faced with children and families from a diverse culture is to maintain an attitude of openness and respectful curiosity, and a willingness to question our own cultural assumptions (Coward and Dattani, 1993, Kemps 1997, Harper and Dwivedi 2004; Maitra, in press).

Conclusions

1   The way childhood is conceptualised in a culture shapes the experiences and development of a child's emotional and relational repertoires.

2   The fact that Indian value systems are not based on the dichotomous systems central to Western thought (such as individual/collective, man/nature, body/mind) make these no less valid. It does mean, however, that much more exploration is necessary of the contexts within which its values are situated before understanding is possible.

3   Characteristics such as interdependence, interpersonal harmony and co-operation, non-verbal and indirect communication, appear to be more highly valued in Indian and in other Eastern cultures (Dwivedi, 2002; Lau, 2002). These cultures may be wary, if not frankly critical, of the value placed by modern Western cultures on individualism, and of the priority given to individual needs above those of hierarchies and groups.

4   The goals of child development are influenced by how a culture constructs the meaning and purpose of life. The Hindu tradition considers mortal existence an opportunity to accumulate good *karma* in order to attain *moksha*, the liberation from the cycle of birth and re-birth. This lingers in contemporary Indian thought as an ideal, encouraging non-attachment and creating an ambivalence towards material possessions and worldly status.

5   Beliefs about *karma* and *moksha* also influence contemporary Indian attitudes towards imperfection, disease and misfortune, encouraging acceptance rather than the motivation to allocate blame, or to seek control or redress. While this may contribute to passivity, at its best it leads to resilience in the face of adversity.

6   The rapid and increasing exposure to global influences may expose children and young people (whether living in India or growing up outside it) to conflict between contradictory value systems. This may contribute to innovative solutions and hybrid cultural forms, or sometimes create vulnerability, leading to maladaptive behaviour or mental health problems.

---

[14] For example, the stereotyped ways in which Asian cultures are mentioned in connection with 'forced marriage' or other oppressions of women, or as family 'pressures'.

7   A useful orientation to cultural diversity would see it as a wealth of solutions devised over centuries to address human dilemmas. This would avoid the insidious damage caused by placing cultural groups in hierarchical positions. While the harm caused by labelling cultures as 'primitive' or 'civilised' seems obvious, similar difficulties arise from the polarisation of 'dominant' and 'minority' cultures. An understanding of how cultural practices are formed allows them to used as therapeutic tools to address similar dilemmas in contemporary contexts.

8   Cross cultural practice requires that professionals maintain an attitude of curiosity leavened with humility when faced with other worldviews, beliefs and value systems.

The authors would like to thank Mary Battison and Karen Amos for help with typing and Kristi Smith for help with literature searches.

References

Banhatti, R. and Bhate, S. (2002): 'Mental health needs of ethnic minority children.' In: K.N. Dwivedi (ed.) *Meeting the Needs of Ethnic Minority Children: A handbook for professionals.* London: Jessica Kingsley Publishers.

Bhagwat, B. K. (2002): Foreword to: *Child Care in Ancient India from the Perspectives of Developmental Psychology and Paediatrics.* By: Kapur, M. and Mukundan, H. Delhi: Sri Satguru Publications.

de Bary, W.T., Hay, S., Weiler, R. and Yarrow, A. (1958) *Sources of Indian Tradition.* New York: Columbia University Press.

Cantile, A. (2003) Myth Text and Context. In V. Das (ed) *The Oxford India Companion to Sociology and Social Anthropology.* Vol 1. p 827-860. Oxford University Press.

Coward, B. and Dattani, P. (1993) 'Race, identity and culture' in Dwivedi K.N. (Ed) *Group Work with Children and Adolescents: A Handbook,* London. Jessica Kingsley

Deivasigamani, T.R. (1990):'Psychiatric morbidity in primary school children: An epidemiological study. *Indian Journal of Psychiatry, 32 (3), 235-40*

Dwivedi, K.N. (1990). 'Purification of Mind by Vipassana Meditation'. In: J. Crook and D. Fontana (Eds.) *Space in Mind.* Shaftesbury. Elements, Chapter 7: 86-91.

Dwivedi, K.N. (Ed.) (1997) *The Therapeutic Use of Stories.* London: Routledge.

Dwivedi, K.N. (Ed.) (2000) *Post Traumatic Stress Disorder in Children and Adolescents.* London: Whurr.

Dwivedi, K.N. (2002) 'Culture and Personality', in Dwivedi, K.N. (Ed.) *Meeting the Needs of Ethnic Minority Children.* 2nd Edition. London: Jessica Kingsley

Dwivedi, K.N. (2004) 'Emotion regulation and mental health' in Dwivedi, K.N. & Harper, P.B. (Eds) *Promoting Emotional Well Being of Children and Adolescents and Preventing their Mental Ill Health: A Handbook.* London: Jessica Kingsley.

Dwivedi, K.N. & Gardner, D. (1997) 'Theoretical perspectives and clinical approaches', in Dwivedi, K.N. (Ed.) *The Therapeutic Use of Stories.* London: Routledge.

Dwivedi, K.N. and Prasad, K.M.R. (2000): The Hindu, Jain and Buddhist communities: beliefs and practices. In: Lau (ed.) *South Asian Children and Adolescents in Britain.* London: Whurr.

Dwivedi, K.N. & Varma, V.P. (Eds) (1997) *Depression in Children and Adolescents.* London: Whurr.

Guha, R. (ed) (1982) 'Preface'. *In Subaltern Studies I.* Delhi: Oxford University Press.

Hackett, L. and Hackett, R. (1993) Parental ideas of normal and deviant child behaviour: A comparison of two ethnic groups. *British Journal of Psychiatry 162,* 353-357.

Harper, P.B. and Dwivedi, R. (2004) 'Developing culturally sensitive services to meet the mental health needs of ethnic minority children' in Dwivedi, K.N. & Harper, P.B. (Eds) *Promoting Emotional Well Being of Children and Adolescents and Preventing their Mental Ill Health: A Handbook.* London: Jessica Kingsley.

Hofstede, G. (1991): *Cultures and Organisations: Softwares of the Mind.* New York: McGraw Hill.

Joshi, M.S. and MacLean, M., (1997): 'Maternal expectations of child development in India, Japan and England.' *Journal of Cross Cultural Psychology, 28, 219-234.*

Kakar, S. (1982) *Shamans, Mystics and Doctors: A Psychological Inquiry into India and its Healing Traditions.* Delhi: OUP.

Kakar, S. (1997): *The Inner World-a Psychoanalytic Study of Childhood and Society in India.* Second edition: Ninth impression. Delhi: Oxford University Press.

Kapur, M., Barnabus, I., Reddy, M. V., Rozario, J. and Uma, H. (1995) *Developmental Psychopathology Check List for Children.* A preliminary report, NIMHANS Journal, 13, (1), 1-9.

Kapur, M., U. H., Reddy, M.V., Barnabus, I.P., and Singhal, D. (1997): 'Study of infant temperament: An Indian perspective', *Indian Journal of Clinical Psychology, 24 (2), 171-177.*

Kemps, C.R. (1997) 'Approaches to working with ethnicity and culture' in Dwivedi, K.N. (Ed.) *Enhancing Parenting Skills.* Chichester: John Wiley

Kumar, K. (1993) Study of childhood and family. In T.S. Saraswathi and Baljit Kaur (eds) *Human Development and Family Studies in India: An agenda for research and policy,* p 67-76. New Delhi: Sage Publications.

Lau A. (2002): 'Family therapy and ethnic minorities', in Dwivedi K.N. (Ed.) *Meeting the Needs of Ethnic Minority Children'.* London: Jessica Kingsley publishers.

Lokare, V. (1997) 'Cultural aspects of anxiety in children' in Dwivedi, K.N. & Varma, V.P. (Eds) *A Handbook of Childhood Anxiety Mangagement.* Aldershot: Arena Publishers.

Lynch, O.M. (1990) 'The social construction of emotion in India', in O.M. Lynch (Ed.) *Divine Passions: The social construction of emotion in India.* California: University of California Press

Madan, T.N. (2003) Religions in India Plurality and Pluralism. In V. Das (ed) *The Oxford India Companion to Sociology and Social Anthropology.* Vol 1. p 775-801. Oxford University Press.

Maitra, B. (1995) Giving due consideration to families racial and cultural backgrounds. In P. Reder and C. Lucey (Eds) *Assessment of Parenting: Psychiatric and Psychological Considerations.* London: Routledge.

Maitra, B. (2004) 'The cultural relevance of mental health disciplines' in M. Malek and C. Joughin (Eds) *Mental Health Services for Minority Ethnic Children and Adolescents.* London: Jessica Kingsley Publishers.

Maitra, B. (in press) The many cultures of child protection. In (ed) Lee Combrinck Graham.

Maitra, B. and Miller, A. (2002) Children, families and therapists: clinical considerations and ethnic minority cultures. In (Eds) K.N. Dwivedi and V.P. Varma – *Meeting the Needs of Ethnic Minority Children – A handbook for professionals.* Second Edition. London: Jessica Kingsley.

Malhotra, S. (1995): 'Study of psychosocial correlates of developmental psychopathology in school children'. Report submitted to the Indian Council for Medical Research, New Delhi.

Markus, H. and Kitayama, S. (1991) 'Culture and self: Implications for cognition, emotion and motivation'. *Psychological Review, 98, 224-253.*

Meltzer, H., Gatward, R., Goodman, R. and Ford, T. (2000) *Mental Health of Children and Adolescents in Great Britain.* London: The Stationary Office.

Nandy, A. (1999): *The intimate enemy: loss and recovery of self under colonialism.* Delhi: Oxford University Press.

Nederveen Pieterse, J. and Parekh, B. (1995) *The Decolonization of Imagination: Culture, Knowledge, and Power.* London and Atlantic Highlands: Zed Books.

Rogoff, B., Sellers, M.J., Pirrotta, S., Fox, N. and White, S.H. (1975) Age of assignment of roles and responsibilities to children A cross-cultural survey. *Human Development,* 18: 353-369.

Roland, A. (1980) 'Psychoanalytic perspectives on personality development in India'. *International Review of Psychoanalysis,* 1, 73-87

Saumarez-Smith, R. (2003) The historiography of Indian society. In V. Das (ed) *The Oxford India Companion to Sociology and Social Anthropology.* Vol 1, p 99-114. New Delhi: Oxford University Press.

Thapar, R. (1966) *A History of India.* Vol 1. London: Penguin Books.

Thomas, A. and Chess, S. (1977): *Temperament and Development.* Brunner/Mazel. New York.

Uberoi, P. (2003) The Family in India Beyond the Nuclear versus Joint Debate. In V. Das (ed) *The Oxford India Companion to Sociology and Social Anthropology.* Vol 2, p 1061-1103. New Delhi: Oxford University Press.

5
Childhood trauma as a cause of ADHD, aggression, violence and anti-social behaviour

Charles Whitfield

Behaviour problems, aggression and violence have increased recently to become a more visible national and international problem. These toxic behaviours are often a component of various mental and behavioural disorders, including some personality disorders, as exemplified in the extreme by many with antisocial personality disorder, and in some people with alcohol or other drug addictions. They have also been further categorized as constituting a part of other clinical conditions such as conduct disorder, oppositional defiant disorder (ODD), Attention Deficit Hyperactivity Disorder (ADHD) and Attention Deficit Disorder (ADD). Disruptive behaviour disorders are said to effect up to ten per cent of children and as many as a third of those who are referred for psychiatric treatment (Ford, 2002; Ford et al, 1999; 2000).

ADHD and ADD

Whether called attention deficit hyperactivity disorder (ADHD) in children or attention deficit disorder (ADD) in adults, this increasingly identified condition of children by teachers, parents and health-care workers has three main diagnostic criteria, any two of which are said to suffice for making the diagnosis: poor *attention* skills, decreased *impulse* control and *hyperactivity*. (For adults diagnosed with "ADD", usually only their attention is a problem, which may make the diagnosis suspect). Yet critics have noted that there is *no valid laboratory or other test for* ADHD, and there is no convincing evidence that ADHD is caused by a primary brain malfunction or any other biological or genetic abnormality (Diller, 2002; Timimi et al, 2004). But another avenue may be more practical and help in prevention. What do we know about its connection to trauma[1]?

---

[1] Childhood trauma may include any one or a combination of physical abuse, sexual abuse, or psychological (emotional) abuse, or neglect. It may occur in the presence of other life stressors, such as having a chemical dependent or mentally ill parent, frequent family moves, loss of a parent, and multiple family deaths. While trauma may be interpreted differently in different cultures, there is general agreement about its basic definitions and that it is common (Ross, 2000; Whitfield, 2003; 2004).

History 1

John was a six year old boy who was diagnosed with ADHD by his schoolteacher and referring paediatrician. He was prescribed the stimulant drug methylphenidate (Ritalin), which helped his symptoms minimally and intermittently. His parents had separated two years previously and were fighting for custody. John's mother came to me for assistance, describing John's symptoms and situation, which indicated that he may have been physically and/or sexually abused by his paternal grandfather. John's symptoms included a pattern of his having insomnia, nightmares, and hyper-irritability for a week or more after each visit with his grandfather. I reported John's symptoms and my concerns to the appropriate local Child Protective Services, which on follow-up did not complete their investigation. His father continued to let John's grandfather see him alone, after which John continued to be upset, clingy and had nightmares. After his grandfather died 11 months later, John's symptoms gradually improved. He is now symptom free.

John's frightening and sad story illustrates a common pattern among children diagnosed with ADHD and given Ritalin or other stimulants. The child's parents are often in conflict and may abuse or neglect the child. As a response, the child "acts out" or has a behaviour problem in and out of school, and the teacher inappropriately labels the child with ADHD and refers him to a physician who prescribes a stimulant drug. Even if someone tries to intervene to protect the child from abuse or neglect, the dysfunctional parental-educational-health care system in which he becomes stuck cannot or does not provide or allow the needed protection.

Substitute almost any other childhood mental disorder for ADHD and we may see that this same pattern is repeated for countless traumatized children. Many of the more than 300 data based studies that I have described in *The Truth About Depression* and *The Truth About Mental Illness* (Whitfield 2003b; 2004), have evaluated children with some of these "mental disorders" and found that a significant percentage of them had been abused or neglected. Their results indicate and their authors recommended that *all children with mental or behavioural symptoms, problems or disorders should be carefully screened and followed for a history of past and present childhood trauma* (Whitfield 2003a; 2004).

History 2

After eighteen months into his participation in trauma-focussed group therapy, Ralph, a successfully recovering alcoholic, thought he might have adult ADD and found a health professional who specialised in treating people with the disorder. As expected, the specialist diagnosed adult ADD and referred Ralph to a psychiatrist who worked in the same clinic and who prescribed a potent stimulant drug, which he tried for several weeks with no improvement in his symptoms of difficulty concentrating and occasional impulsiveness. He told us later in group, "I thought I had ADD and wanted to have it in case a stimulant might help me calm down and focus on my work or whatever else I needed to do. But the drugs didn't help and now, a year later, I realise that I was looking for a short cut around my grieving. I had to try it anyway, to realise that I can do better without drugs, through my work on the effects of my past trauma here in group and in individual counselling and AA".

Ralph got off easy. Three other patients of mine did not. Also recovering chemical dependents, they went the same route as did Ralph (believing they had ADD), but got addicted to the Ritalin for two to five years, respectively, during which time it actually made their ADD symptoms of difficulty concentrating and low energy worse, instead of better. It took them more than two years of bothersome stimulant withdrawal symptoms to finally stop taking Ritalin. They were also severely psychologically abused as children, but elected not to confront their trauma wounds at that time.

Causal Factors

These example case histories do not mean that: 1) all children and adults with symptoms and signs of ADHD/ADD do not have it, 2) they will become harmfully involved with the stimulant drugs in treatment, or 3) they have a history of childhood trauma. But many who are erroneously diagnosed with ADHD/ADD – and some who are accurately diagnosed with it – may have one or more of these crucial characteristics. I believe all people with symptoms or signs of ADHD/ADD should be evaluated for a history of trauma.

Other conditions can stimulate the symptoms and signs of ADHD/ADD, including Post Traumatic Stress Disorder (PTSD), heavy alcohol or other drug use and other mental illness – all of which should be excluded first. Poor to marginal nutrition, including eating many sugar products and other processed and junk food and caffeine can cause and aggravate ADHD symptoms. Finally, a troubled or stressful environment can do the same. A primary question here is: How does childhood trauma relate to this only-recently described disorder?

Retrospective and Prospective Study Evidence

I found 77 published reports of a significantly higher incidence of ADHD among abused children. Fifteen of these were from *prospective* studies and 58 were *retrospective*, as shown in Table 5.1. These investigations were conducted on a total of 168,801 traumatised children – and adults with a history of it – and their controls. 17 of these 77 studies looked for and found ADHD, and 49 of them did not look specifically for ADHD (for various reasons) but found behaviour problems, school problems and delinquency, while 7 found oppositional defiant disorder and 8 found conduct disorder. Thus, most of these studies did not look specifically for ADHD but found behavioural signs of it. In fact, most of the other studies on traumatized children referred to throughout *The Truth About Depression* and *The Truth About Mental Illness* (Whitfield 2003b; 2004) didn't look for ADHD, possibly because this disorder was not as prominent at the time these studies were conducted. I found only one study that looked for it that reported a negative association of ADD with trauma (Wozniak et al, 1999). These data are impressive enough to support including trauma as an aggravating or causal factor to be addressed clinically, and its extent warrants further research. Another factor, low self-esteem, is common, if not usual among people with ADHD/ADD.

Index Cases [2]

For index case studies, relatively fewer people with diagnosed ADHD and other problematic behaviour, including violence, have been evaluated for a history of childhood trauma. I found four reports for children diagnosed with ADHD. These involved 436 children and teens with ADHD and/or oppositional defiant disorder (ODD) and their controls (i.e. children with neither of these disorders). Those who had these disorders and behaviours had a significantly higher history of childhood trauma than their controls or the general population. There was also more associated PTSD and other co-morbidity. The authors concluded that there was a need to address trauma in most children with behaviour problems.

---

[2] An 'Index case' is a person who is diagnosed with ADHD, ADD, or any other disorder under study.

Table 5.1.

ADHD, behaviour problems and childhood trauma: Clinical, community, prospective, index case studies, and meta-analysis/literature reviews.

Year/study	Sample	ADHD/ Behaviour problems	Other trauma effects
Clinical/community 58 studies 1937-2003	153,185 people CT v. Controls	Increased to 15x controls	Increase co-morbidity
Prospective studies 15 studies 1996-2003	15,227 people CT v. Controls	Increased to 16x controls	Increase co-morbidity
Index 4 studies 1999-2000	389 children with ADHD and their controls	Increased to 73% with a CT history	Increase co-morbidity
Meta-analysis/ Literature reviews 1989-2001	2 literature reviews and 1 meta-analysis	Increased association with CT among all	Increase co-morbidity
Summary 77 studies by independent international authors 1985-2003	168,801 CT people and controls	Increased link between CT and ADHD/behaviour problems Increased to 15x clinical/community Increased to 3.2x prospective Increased to 73% CT in index cases	Increase co-morbidity All document CT link

Key:
CT = childhood trauma

Multiple co-morbidity is a marker of the advanced effects of childhood trauma (Felitti et al, 1998; Ross, 2000; Whitfield, 2003; 2004). The fact that children with ADHD are at high risk for multiple disorders and conditions, such as PTSD, depression, substance abuse, chemical dependence, school problems and dropout, low self-esteem, teen pregnancy, and others, further suggests that there may be a significant link between trauma and ADHD.

If a child or adult who is diagnosed with ADHD or ADD has experienced repeated trauma, they may also have PTSD. In fact, if their teacher, school counsellor, physician or parent is not knowledgeable about PTSD, they may have misdiagnosed ADHD/ADD when they actually have PTSD or have it in addition to ADHD. The symptoms and signs of these two disorders are similar, and PTSD can easily be mistaken for ADHD/ADD, as shown in Table 5.2.

Table 5.2

Differential diagnosis of ADHD and PTSD- similarities

ADHD Category	PTSD diagnostic criteria
Inattention	Acting or feeling as if the trauma were recurring. Distress at exposure to cues resembling the trauma. Re-experiencing trauma. Problems concentrating. Hyper-vigilant to perceived fear stimuli. Avoiding stimuli associated with trauma.
Hyperactivity/Impulsivity	Acting or feeling as if trauma were recurring. Distress at exposure to cues resembling the trauma. Inability to appropriately inhibit hyper-vigilance. Psychological reactivity when exposed to cues symbolizing the trauma. Irritability and anger outbursts.
Externalizing behaviours	Acting or feeling as if trauma were recurring. Distress at exposure to cues resembling the trauma. Avoiding activities, people or places. Markedly diminished interest/participation in activities. Feeling detached. Restricted range of affect. Exaggerated startle response. Repetitive play with trauma themes. Irritability and anger outbursts.

If a child or adult with PTSD is misdiagnosed as having ADHD or ADD and treated with stimulant drugs, their symptoms may get worse, which I have observed among several of my patients. In such a case, the physician may erroneously try to increase the dose or switch to another stimulant or other psychoactive drug. There are several other drawbacks. Such misdiagnoses and mistreatment may only re-traumatise the person. As the family medicine physician, Anna Kirkengen (2001), said, "Every time we deny a trauma survivor's reality, we re-victimise them".

Behaviour problems in general are common among abused and neglected children. For example, Calam and colleagues (1998) reported a significant increase in behaviour and attentional problems among 144 sexually abused children followed for two years. The children were evaluated initially, and then at one, nine, and twenty-four months later. The research team found an increase in fifteen other problems over the two year follow up. These findings are impressive, since they show how abused and neglected children are hurt by trauma, and yet are often *misdiagnosed* or even *blamed for having* these *trauma-induced results* (Calam et al, 1998). Rather than address these effects appropriately as being caused by the trauma, many authority figures such as parents, teachers, law enforcement people, and some clinicians commonly label and blame the child, which re-victimizes them further and decreases their already low self-esteem (see Table 5.3).

Table 5.3

Problems found among sexually abused children (in percentage).
Followed 2 years, in order of decreasing frequency (from Calam et al 1998)

Disturbance/problem	1 month	9 months	2 years
School difficulties	18	29	39
Attention problems	11	20	33
Sleep problems	20	34	33
Anger	10	34	33
Anxiety/depression	19	36	31
Sexualized behaviour	11	28	23
Somatic complaints	11	16	18
Eating problems	7	9	17
Lack peer relationships	3	25	15
Wetting and soiling	11	18	15
Running away	8	11	13
Substance abuse	2	5	10
Suicide attempts	0	4	8
Self-mutilation	0	5	5
Speech problems	5	5	2
Clumsiness	2	5	1

How helpful is it to label children with new 'disorders' such as 'ADHD' when, instead, the child's behaviour may be a normal reaction to an abnormal environment? The child's dysfunctional educational system, teachers, parents and exposure to toxic media may be a major part of the problem. Child psychiatrist Sami Timimi and 33 co-endorsers (Including myself) published a critique (Timimi et al, 2004) of the current party-line view of ADHD as espoused in an 'International Consensus Statement' by long-time ADHD advocate Russell Barkley and co-endorsers (Barkley et al, 2002).

Citing the above concerns in our critique, we noted there were no valid diagnostic tests or brain abnormalities for this claimed disorder, and that there were no studies that showed that Ritalin/stimulants were helpful in the long term. We also noted that ADHD is mostly a cultural construct to cover up a dysfunctional educational and parenting system. Rather than engage us in a healthy debate, Barkley et al. answered with platitudes that essentially translated that they had the truth about ADHD, while we did not (Barkley et al, 2004).

Paediatrician Lawrence Diller noted that: 1) over half of children receiving Ritalin do not have ADHD; 2) Ritalin/stimulants are not specific for ADHD. They increase everyone's ability to focus. But they do not help parents parent or teachers teach any better; and 3) while our culture benefits from diversity, we train our children to think and behave the same, and if they don't, we give them Ritalin (Diller, 2002).

Psychologist Diane Willis said, "When we consider the reasons behind the current trend in medicating young children, parents, physicians, and even psychologists must bear some of the responsibility. Parents often do not choose psychological interventions over medications because of the extra demands on their time to participate in therapy or bring their child for therapy. The expense of psychological interventions is measured in terms of time demands as well as professional and clinic fees, and busy parents may be unwilling to devote the effort to weekly sessions and/or practice new management techniques with their child. Parents may also consider a medically treatable diagnosis to be less of a personal reflection on their parenting skills or their own characteristics, and therefore less stigmatizing. When parents ask their child's physician for treatment suggestions, there is pressure on the physician to address parents' concerns immediately, and prescribing medication is often the result. However, the least expensive approach to managing a young child's behaviour (i.e., medication) may end up, in the long run, being the most costly. If we look at who is doing the medicating, it is often general practitioners and paediatricians rather than mental health professionals such as child psychiatrists." (Willis, 2003).

In figure 5.1 I outline an approach to recognizing and treating a child with behaviour problems suggestive of ADHD, oppositional defiant disorder or conduct disorder.

Figure 5.1

ADHD, ODD, CD: Flowchart for decision making.

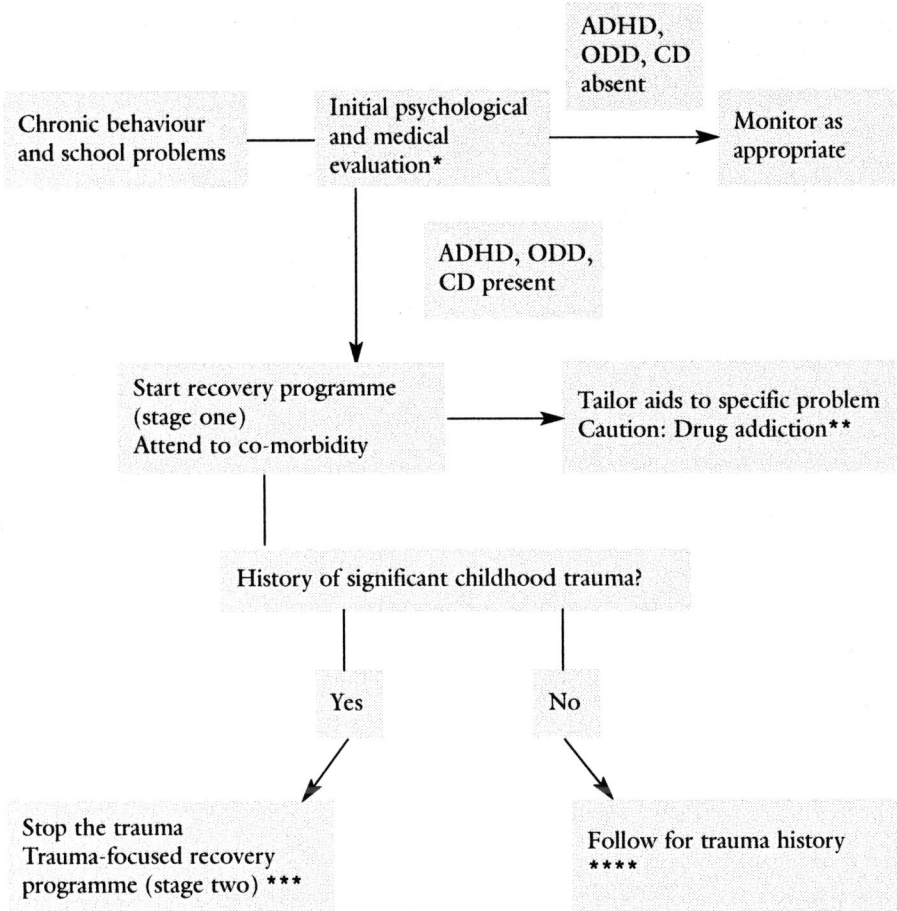

*   Rule out more complex forms or causes of behaviour/school problems e.g. addiction, dissociative states, serious physical problem and other effects of childhood trauma.
**   Avoid using drugs to treat children, including stimulants and especially benzodiazepine sedative drugs to treat anxiety, insomnia or depression. SSRIs are dangerous and ineffective for children and adolescents.
***   Family therapy, group and individual therapy, self-help groups for parents.
****   Because many trauma survivors authentically forget the trauma (dissociative amnesia), or they may not be able to accurately name what happened to them as having been traumatic, or are embarrassed or want to protect the parents, keep an open mind that a substantial number of these people may eventually disclose a serious trauma.

Aggression, violence and anti-social behaviour

Most children and adults with ADHD and ADD are neither harmfully aggressive, violent nor antisocial. But these inappropriate behaviours may be part of a pattern, as explored and found in 38 clinical and community studies and sixteen prospective ones that reported an association between these toxic behaviours and having a history of childhood trauma.

Retrospective studies

I found 38 clinical and community sample studies conducted by independent research teams over the last three decades between the 1970s and 2000 that evaluated 45,088 traumatized children and adults with that history, and their controls. They all found a significant link between childhood trauma and subsequent aggressive and violent behaviour, with odds ratio (risk factors) as high as four times that for the controls. These 38 studies are but the tip of the iceberg regarding the firm link between childhood trauma and people's subsequent acting out of violence.

Prospective studies

I found 16 prospective studies that followed traumatized children and their controls for up to 19 years. All showed a statistically significant link between having a history of repeated childhood trauma and subsequent aggressive behaviour and violence, with odds ratios of up to 22 times that for controls.

Index case studies

I found 6 studies of severely aggressive or violent people that reported a significantly high percentage (up to 100 percent) of them having had a history of repeated childhood trauma.

Table 5.4

Aggression violence and childhood trauma: Clinical and community, prospective, index case studies

Year/study	Sample	Aggression and violence	Other trauma effects
Clinical and community 38 studies 1977-2003	45,088 people CT v. controls	Increased aggressive and/or violent behaviour	Increased co-morbidity
Prospective 16 studies 1990-2003	8,277 people CT v. controls	Increased to 22x	Decreased self-esteem Increase co-morbidity
Index case 10 studies 1982-2003	927 ADHD, ODD or violent children	Increased to 100% had CT history	Increased co-morbidity
Summary 64 studies by independent international authors 1977-2003	54,242 people	Increased link between CT and aggression and/or violence	Increased co-morbidity

Key:
CT – childhood trauma

Summary

These add up to a total of 64 studies by independent researchers using multiple study designs on 54,242 people in different countries that show a highly significant relationship between repeated childhood trauma and later aggressive or violent behaviour (Table 5.4). This is impressive evidence that clinicians, parents, teachers and others should take into account in their work, especially regarding prevention of further violence. In the next section I will review selected examples from these 66 studies, after which I will review some important dynamics relating to family and gender issues.

Example studies

Whether treating children violently is likely to make them treat others violently later in life is of great social importance. In an attempt to sort out whether violence breads violence across generations, in 1989 researcher Cathy Widom analyzed 18 reports on the topic published from 1970 to 1986 and said that there were not enough data to draw any firm conclusions at that time. But more recent studies have shown that maltreated children are at risk for many psychological, behavioural, and physical problems including aggression and violence, as I have described elsewhere (Whitfield 2003a; 2004; Whitfield et al, 2003).

Three examples include: 1) Shields and Cicchetti (1998) measured the effects of childhood trauma on 141 abused, inner-city children who they compared with 87 controls. They found that the abused children exhibited increased levels of violent, aggressive behaviour, especially those who were physically abused. Other effects of the trauma included increased emotional swings, dissociation, and difficulty focusing, all of which simulate ADHD (Shields and Cicchetti, 1998; 2001).

2) Another research group looked at 4,790 middle- and high-schoolers and found higher levels of anti-social behaviour, as well as more substance abuse and suicidal behaviour, among those who self-reported having been abused, than was found among controls (Bensley et al, 1999; 2000).

3) Widom and colleagues followed 1,575 abused children long-term, and published their findings in five reports (see Widom and Shepard, 1996; Widom and Morris, 1997; Widom, 1999). They found that abused children had more aggression, violence and anti-social behaviour, as well as an increased risk of depression, suicide, anxiety, substance abuse and PTSD than did the control children. Numerous others have found similar results (Whitfield et al, 2003) and they provide firm evidence for such a link.

Family and gender dynamics

Research on the transgenerational transmission of family aggression and violence began 40 years ago (MacEwen, 1994). Multiple factors are often at play. These factors may include the type of abuse, and whether it was experienced, witnessed or both; its severity and frequency; the victim's identification with and imitation of the abuser and/or other victims; enabling behaviour (co-abuse) by others; gender identification; the overall impact of the trauma(s); self-esteem (shame) of the victim; memory of the trauma; the use of survival defences; and the recovery process itself (Archer, 2000; MacEwen, 1994; Whitfield et al, 2001; Whitfield, 1995).

The abused person's current adult relationships add more factors: the trauma history of the partner; the partner's current behaviour; the interpersonal dynamics and boundaries of the current relationship (Whitfield, 1993); and the abused person's attachment history in infancy and later (Lyons-Ruth and Jacobvitz, 1999) Other factors, such as repeated viewing of TV and movie violence, contribute to and aggravate the cycle.

Women and men can be either victims or perpetrators of violence (Archer, 2000; Archer and Ray, 1989; Fergusson et al, 1996; 2000; Henton et al, 1993; Magdol et al, 1997; Sets and Strauss, 1989). Each gender appears to initiate the violence with equal frequency. However, women are more likely than men to suffer injuries as a victim and men more likely to be perpetrators of the injuries (Archer, 2000; Fergusson and Horwood, 1998). Archer (2000) did a meta-analysis of eighty-two separate reports of aggression among partners. He found that while women use physical aggression on men about as often as do men on women, more women than men reported having been injured (62 versus 38 percent, respectively). This process is often related to the phenomenon of subsequent re-victimization as adults for people who were abused as children.

Exposure to violence by witnessing it is also traumatic. For example, Hurt and colleagues (2001) studied 119 inner-city children who had a high exposure to violence by age seven years, and found significant signs of distress that frequently were not recognized by caregivers. Among the children, 75 percent had heard gunshots, 60 percent had seen drug deals, 18 percent had seen a dead body outside, and 10 percent had seen a shooting or stabbing happen in the home. Higher exposure to violence in children was linked with poorer school performance, symptoms of anxiety and depression and lower self-esteem, some of which could be misdiagnosed and mistreated as having 'ADHD'.

These findings – that children exposed to abuse and violence are at increased risk of interpersonal violence later in life – have implications for personal recovery, clinical practice and prevention. Clinicians should screen for a history of violence and victimization in both men and women, as well as for a history of childhood trauma itself (Briere, 1996; Courtois, 1991; Whitfield et al, 2003; Whitfield, 1995; 2003a and b). By making these connections and offering effective treatment or referral, we can assist in all levels of prevention. We have to stop abusing and neglecting our children.

Becoming involved in violence either as a victim *or* a perpetrator is a high-risk behaviour. In the ongoing adverse childhood experiences (ACE) study, Rob Anda, Vince Felitti, and their colleagues have now evaluated over 17,000 adults regarding their trauma, medical and behavioural histories (Anda et al, in press; Felitti et al, 1998; Whitfield et al, 2003; Whitfield, 2004). Based on their findings, they have proposed and shown how repeated childhood trauma (ACEs) lead to a multitude of health and social problems that result from disrupted development of the brain and nervous system. This disrupted neurodevelopment then is significantly related to impairment in the victim's social, emotional and cognitive (thinking and remembering) functioning, which causes or aggravates the adoption of high-risk behaviours. These high-risk behaviours are many and varied such as overeating, heavy alcohol and other drug use (including nicotine), sexual promiscuity and other kinds of self-harm. Less commonly known, becoming involved in violence in any way is also highly risky, as are not wearing seat belts, not exercising or maintaining oral hygiene. These high-risk behaviours then lead to an increase in disease, disability and social problems, which in turn can cause early death, as shown in Figure 5.2. These detrimental effects of childhood trauma can be prevented in most of these levels in this pyramid by appropriate intervention by individuals or their clinicians.

Figure 5.2

Mechanisms by which adverse childhood experiences influence health and well-being throughout the lifespan.

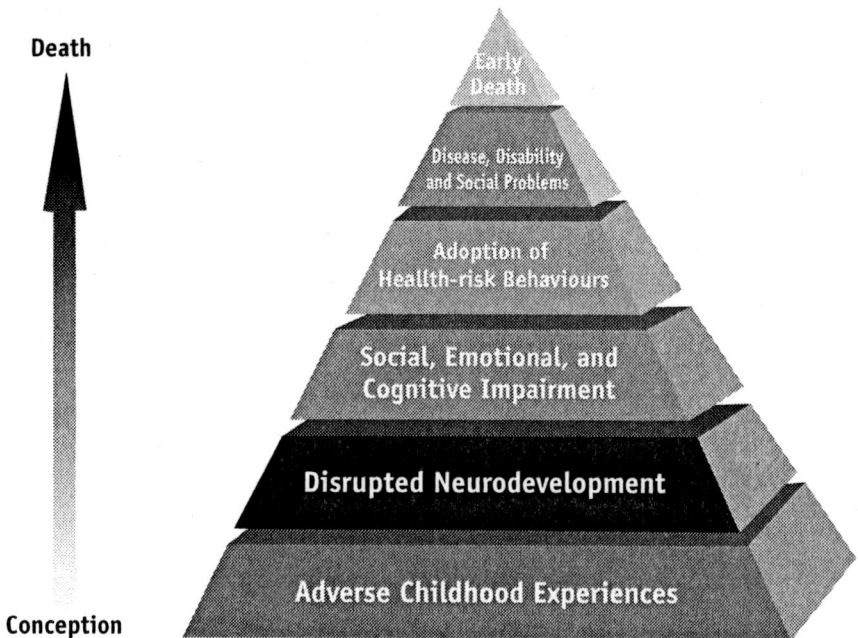

Death

Early Death

Disease, Disability and Social Problems

Adoption of Heallth-risk Behaviours

Social, Emotional, and Cognitive Impairment

Disrupted Neurodevelopment

Adverse Childhood Experiences

Conception

Mechanisms by Which Adverse Childhood Experiences
Influence Health and Well-being Throughout the Lifespan

While anyone can be aggressive and violent, among the most common disorders associated with them are alcohol and other drug addiction, antisocial personality disorder and psychoses. Cigarette smokers commonly use nicotine to help hold down their anger. Many of the hundreds of research reports linking childhood trauma to subsequent mental illness found inordinate anger to be a significant long-term effect of repeated childhood trauma.

Aggression and violence are the toxic end result of inordinate and unhandled anger. Clinical psychologist, Ron Potter-Efron, has written a helpful workbook on anger management (Potter-Efron and Potter-Efron, 1995) and I have a section that begins to address it in *A Gift to Myself* (Whitfield, 1991). It is useful to view anger as part of the normal and healthy process of grieving from childhood and other trauma, and to learn safe and effective ways to prevent it from escalating to aggression and violence.[3]

---

[3] The full list references for of all studies summarized in this chapter can be found in Whitfield C.L.: *The Truth about Mental Illness.* Choices for Healing. Health Communications, Deerfield Beach, FL, 2004.

References

Anda, R.F., Felitti, V.J., Walker, J., Whitfield, C.L., Bremner, J.D., Perry, B.D., Dube, S.R. and Giles, W.H. (2004) The enduring effects of childhood abuse and related experiences: a convergence of evidence from neurobiology and epidemiology (in press).

Archer, J. (2000) Sex differences in aggression between heterosexual partners: A meta-analytic review. *Psychological Bulletin* 126, 651-680.

Archer, J. and Ray, N. (1989) Dating violence in the United Kingdom: a preliminary study. *Aggressive Behaviour* 15, 337-343.

Barkley, R.A. et al (2002) International Consensus Statement on ADHD. *Clinical Child and Family Psychology Review* 5, 89- 111.

Barkley, R.A. et al (2004) Critique or misrepresentation? A reply to Timimi et al. *Clinical Child and Family Psychology Review* 7, 65-69.

Bensley, L.B., Van Eenwyck, J. and Simmons, K.W. (2000) Self-reported childhood sexual and physical abuse and adult HIV-risk behaviours and heavy drinking. *American Journal of Preventive Medicine* 18, 151-158.

Bensley, L.B., Speiker, S.J., Van Eenwyck, J. and Schoder, J. (1999) Self-reported abuse history and adolescent problem behaviours. 1. Antisocial and suicidal behaviours. *Journal of Adolescent Health* 24, 163-172.

Brier, J.N. (1996) *Treatment of Adults Sexually Molested as Children: Beyond Survival (Rev. 2nd ed.)*. New York: Springer.

Calam, R.M., Horne, L., Glasgow, D. and Cox, A. (1998) Psychological disturbance in child sexual abuse: a follow-up study. *Child Abuse and Neglect* 22, 901-913.

Courtois, C. (1991) Theory, sequencing and strategy in treating adult survivors. In J. Brier (ed.) *Treating Victims of Child Sexual Abuse*. Jossey-Bass.

Diller, L.H. (2002) Prescription stimulant use in American children: Ethical issues. *PCBE*, 12th Dec.

Felitti, V.J., Anda, R.F., Nordenberg, D., Williamson, D.F., Spitz, A.M., Edwards, V., Koss, M.P. and Marks, J.S. (1998) Relationship of childhood abuse and household dysfunction to many leading causes of death in adults. *American Journal of Preventive Medicine* 14, 245-258.

Fergusson, D.M. and Horwood, L.I. (1998) Exposure to interpersonal violence in childhood and psychological dysfunction in young adulthood. *Child Abuse and Neglect* 22, 339-357.

Fergusson, D.M., Horwood, L.I. and Lynskey, M.T. (1996) Childhood sexual abuse and psychiatric disorder in young adulthood: II. Psychiatric outcomes of childhood sexual abuse. *Journal of the American Academy of Child and Adolescent Psychiatry* 34, 1365-1374.

Fergusson, D.M., Horwood, L.I. and Woodward, L.J. (2000) The stability of child abuse reports: A longitudinal study of the reporting behaviour of young adults. *Psychological Medicine* 30, 529-544.

Ford, J.D. (2002) Traumatic victimization in childhood and persistent problems with oppositional-defiance. *Journal of Trauma, Maltreatment and Aggression* 11, 25-58,

Ford, J.D., Racusin, R., Daviss, W.B., Ellis, C.G., Thomas, J., Rogers, K., Reiser, J., Schiffman, J. and Sengupta, A. (1999) Trauma Exposure Among Children with Oppositional Defiant Disorder and Attention-Deficit-Hyperactivity Disorder. *Journal of Consultant Clinical Psychology* 67, 786-789.

Ford, J.D., Racusin, R., Ellis, C.G., Daviss, W.B., Reiser, J., Fleischer, A. and Thomas, J. (2000). Child maltreatment, other trauma exposure, and post-traumatic symptomatology among children with oppositional defiant and attention deficit hyperactivity disorders. *Child Maltreatment* 5, 205-217.

Henton, J., Cate, R., Koval, J., Lloyd, S. and Christopher, S. (1993) Romance and violence in dating relationships. *Journal of Family Issues* 4, 467-482.

Hurt, H., Malmud, E., Brodsky, N.L. and Giannetta, J. (2001) Exposure to violence, psychological and academic correlates in child witnesses. *Archives of Pediatric and Adolescent Medicine* 155, 1351-1356.

Kirkengen, A.L. (2001) *Inscribed Bodies: Health Impact of Childhood Sexual Abuse.* Boston: Kluwer Academic.

Lyons-Ruth, K. and Jacobvitz, D. (1999) Attachment disorganization: Unresolved loss, relational violence, and lapses in behavioural and attentional strategies. In J. Cassidy and P.R. Shavers (eds.) *Handbook of attachment: Theory, Research and Clinical Applications.* New York: Guilford Press.

MacEwan, K.E. (1994) Refining the intergenerational transmission hypothesis. *Journal of Interpersonal Violence* 9, 350-365.

Magdol, L., Moffitt, T.E., Caspi, A., Newman, D.L., Fagan, J. and Silva, P.A. (1997) Gender differences in partner violence in a birth cohort of 21-year-olds: Bridging the gap between clinical and epidemiological approaches. *Journal of Consultant Clinical Psychology* 65, 68-77.

Potter-Efron, R. and Potter-Efron, P. (1995) *Letting Go of Anger: The 10 Most Common Anger Styles and What to do About Them.* New York: New Harbinger.

Ross, C.A. (2000) *The Trauma Model: A Solution to the Problem of Co-Morbidity in Psychiatry.* Richardson, TX: Manitou Publications.

Shields, A. and Cicchetti, D. (1998) Reactive aggression among maltreated children: The Contributions of attention and emotion dysregulation. *Journal of Clinical Child Psychology* 27, 381-395.

Shields, A. and Cicchetti, D. (2001) Parental maltreatment and emotion dysregulation as risk factors for bullying and victimization in middle childhood. *Journal of Clinical Child Psychology* 30, 349-363.

Stets, J.E. and Strauss, M.A. (1989) The marriage licence as a hitting licence: A comparison of assaults in dating, co-habiting and married couples. In M.A. Pirog-Good and J.E. Stets (eds.) *Violence in Dating Relationships.* New York: Praeger.

Timimi, S. et al. (2004) A critique of the international consensus statement on ADHD. *Clinical Child and Family Psychology Review* 7, 59-63.

Whitfield, C.L. (1991) *A Gift to Myself.* Deerfield Beach, FL: Health Communications.

Whitfield, C.L. (1993) *Boundaries and Relationships: Knowing, Protecting and Enjoying the Self.* Deerfield Beach, FL: Health Communications.

Whitfield, C.L. (1995) *Memory and Abuse: Remembering and Healing the Wounds of Trauma*. Deerfield Beach, FL: Health Communications.

Whitfield, C.L. (2003a) *My Recovery: A Personal Plan for Healing*. Deerfield Beach, FL: Health Communications.

Whitfield, C.L. (2003b) *The Truth About Depression: Choices for Healing*. Deerfield Beach, FL: Health Communications.

Whitfield, C.L. (2004) *The Truth About Mental Illness: Choices for Healing*. Deerfield Beach, FL: Health Communications.

Whitfield, C.L., Silberg, J. and Fink, P. (2001) Exposing misinformation concerning child sexual abuse and adult survivors. *Journal of Child Sexual Abuse* 9, 1-8.

Whitfield, C.L., Anda, R.F., Dube, S.R. and Felitti, V.J. (2003) Violent childhood experiences and the risk of intimate partner violence in adults: assessment in a large health maintenance organisation. *Journal of Interpersonal Violence* 18, 166-185.

Widom, C.S. (1999) Post-traumatic stress disorder in abused and neglected children grown up. *American Journal of Psychiatry* 156, 1223-1229.

Widom, C.S. and Morris, S. (1997) Accuracy of adult recollections of childhood victimisation: Part 2 – Childhood sexual abuse. *Psychological Assessment* 9, 34-46.

Widom, C.S, and Shepard, R.L. (1996) Accuracy of adult recollections of childhood victimisation: Part 1 – Childhood physical abuse. *Psychological Assessment* 8, 412-421.

Willis, D.J. (2003) The drugging of young children: Why is psychology mute? *The Clinical Psychologist* 56, 1-3.

Wozniak, J., Crawford, M.H., Biederman, J., Faraone, S.V., Spencer, T.J., Taylor, A. and Blier, H.K. (1999) Antecedents and complications of trauma in boys with ADHD: Findings from a longitudinal study. *Journal of the American Academy of Child and Adolescent Psychiatry* 38, 48-55.

6
The truth about academic medicine: Children on psychotropic drugs and the illusion of science

Jonathan Leo

Introduction

"C onfusion, manipulation, and institutional failure" was the recent summary on *The Lancet's* editorial page about the research into selective serotonin reuptake inhibitor (SSRI) use in childhood depression (Editors, 2004). The editors' conclusions were based on revelations that pharmaceutical companies had selectively reported favourable research about the use of antidepressants in children. However, the medical community makes a mistake if it believes that the current problem is just one of unpublished data, which the pharmaceutical companies have kept hidden. If it were only as straightforward as a relatively few acts of corporate irresponsibility, then the solution would be fairly simple, but virtually everyone knows it is more complicated. The SRRIs are not the only drugs involved and, moreover, the pharmaceutical companies are not the only players involved. Forget the companies, with their simplistic slogans about unproven chemical theories of depression. Slogans conveniently interlaced with words like *"maybe,"* *"possibly,"* and *"might"* to ostensibly avoid charges of false advertising by drug regulators. The more important problem is that for ten years the system of academic medicine failed. It failed to the point that the academic journals were circulating a myth about the benefits of psychotropic drugs that had little to do with the truth. However this myth, which states that children in distress or children who do not pay attention in school have diseases requiring medication, is quickly unravelling – faster than most observers could have imagined.

There are numerous examples of how mainstream medicine and its institutions – such as medical schools, medical journals, and government research organizations – have contributed to these myths, yet two cases are especially interesting. One case involves the revelations, which David Healy has brought to light, about the discrepancies between unpublished and published data on antidepressant use in children. The second case relates to clear institutional biases when it comes to the interpretation of data generated from neuroimaging studies comparing medicated ADHD children to unmedicated ADHD children.

Childhood Distress

Marketing Antidepressants

In October 2004, the Food and Drug Administration (FDA) announced that commonly used antidepressants are likely lead to an increase in suicidal thoughts or actions in some children and teens; they also announced that the same problem might exist for adults. Almost one year prior to this, the Medicines and Health Care Products Regulatory Agency (MHRA), the British equivalent of the FDA, effectively banned the use of these drugs, except for Prozac, in children and adolescents less than eighteen years of age. Ten years ago, the market for antidepressants in children was practically non-existent, five years ago, it was booming, and now, it seems to be in jeopardy. Considering how much money we have spent over the past decade on the search for the causes and treatment of mental anguish, who would have thought we would end up with a warning label saying that these drugs might lead to an increased rate of suicide?

In the mid 1980s, adults started to use the selective serotonin reuptake inhibitors (SSRIs) for depression, and since then brand names, such as Prozac, Paxil, and Zoloft, have become entrenched in popular culture. Indeed, three of the seven most commonly used drugs are now mood elevators. By the early 1990s, it didn't matter that they were not officially approved for use in children: they were commonly given to children as young as six years old. In some cases prescriptions were written for infants under twelve months (Grinfeld, 1998).

Although you would never know it from a perusal of the mainstream psychiatry journals over the last decade, when the SSRIs first came on the market in the late 1980s there were hints of increased suicidality in people taking the drugs (Healy, 2003a). It is not surprising that some psychologically distressed people commit suicide; after all, a distressed state is a predisposing factor for suicide. So, naturally, to accusations that the drugs cause some people to take their own lives, the companies' response has always been: It's the disease, not the drug. While it may seem hard to disentangle the role of these two variables, the disease and the drug, there is a way, and it has been done. The place to begin is with the companies' own efficacy studies.

These studies started with a group of depressed patients, which was divided in half. Half the group was given a drug, and the other half a placebo. According to the FDA data, there was an increase in suicidality in the drug-exposed group. Furthermore, this is not an isolated finding, but is the case for almost every single antidepressant studied – in adults, no less (Healy, 2003b). No longer can we simply blame the disease: the drugs appear to be playing a role in making some people more likely to take their lives.

In the late 1990s, the first major scientific papers investigating the use of these drugs in children, funded by the drug companies, started to appear in the medical literature. The studies made a case for these drugs as being safe and effective for the treatment of childhood distress. The studies subsequently became part of the companies' submissions to the FDA to get the drugs approved for children.

However, drug companies do not just supply the FDA with references to published papers, they supply significantly more detail than what is available in the scientific papers. The version submitted to the FDA is not available immediately to the public, but, eventually, some of the data finds its way onto the FDA web site, or becomes available due to court proceedings. Only when all the data is in the public realm, can a comparison between the two versions be made: the one published in the medical literature and the unpublished account submitted to the FDA. It was this embarrassing mismatch between the published and unpublished data that forced the FDA to step back into the fray.

To win approval of a drug, for a given condition, in a certain population, a drug company must submit two positive studies to the FDA. To obtain its two positive studies, the company might do five, six, or as many as ten studies. Even if the majority of the studies are negative, as long as two are positive the drug can be awarded FDA approval. For any given study, the basic idea is that the benefits should outweigh the risks. It is taken for granted that every drug will cause some sort of side effects, but if they are minimal and the benefits are significant, then the FDA, the medical community, and the patients all agree to live with the risks. The FDA considered seven antidepressants for childhood depression (Prozac, Paxil, Zoloft, Celexa, Remeron, Effexor, Serzone), but Prozac was the only drug approved. While *not* approved for the treatment of depression, Zoloft was approved for the treatment of Obsessive Compulsive Disorder (OCD) in children.

Importantly, once a drug is approved, for, perhaps, depression in adults, there is nothing stopping doctors from prescribing the drug to other groups of people – to children, for instance. Nor is there anything to keep doctors from prescribing the drug for other psychiatric conditions, such as, Oppositional Defiant Disorder (ODD). Although Prozac was not approved for children until 2003, it was perfectly legal for doctors to prescribe it, off-label, to children prior to official FDA approval. Likewise, even though the other SSRIs are still not approved for use in children, it is perfectly legal to use them.

In fact, the child psychiatry profession fully endorsed the use of these drugs well before the FDA approved them, and, in an even odder twist, the profession endorsed the use of them well before any of the major studies in children were even published (Koplewicz, 1997). It appears that one reason for doing the studies in the first place was to justify already well-accepted prescribing patterns. If a trend is created "because everyone else is doing it" then it appears that the child psychiatry profession's use of these drugs in the late 1990s more closely resembled a trend instead of a logical scientific undertaking.

How did all this happen? Naturally, there are no easy answers, but, as a start, one needs to look at the studies asserting that these drugs are safe and effective. In the following discussion, the papers written for the scientific community are compared to the FDA documents (Mosholder, 2004). For the most part, the field consists of about 12 papers, spanning almost a decade, which, when stacked together, fit nicely into a three-ring binder. The studies involving the three most common selective serotonin reuptake inhibitors (SSRIs) – Prozac, Paxil, and Zoloft – serve as excellent examples of how, at every step of the way, the benefits were overestimated and the risks underestimated. According to Healy, "*There is probably no other area of medicine in which the academic literature is so at odds with the raw data*" (Healy, 2004: 10). On one hand, debating the details from any one study, about how one or two children's side effects should be categorized, might seem trivial. On the other hand, when the literature on the use of antidepressants in children is looked at, as a complete body of work, there is a problematic track record, which is anything but trivial.

Prozac (Fluoxetine)

The lead author of the two studies submitted to the FDA, as part of Eli Lilly's successful request to get Prozac approved for children was Graham Emslie, a professor at The University of Texas Southwestern Medical Centre at Dallas. The first study, funded by the National Institute of Mental Health (NIMH) and published in 1997, reported that "*Side effects, as a reason for discontinuation, were minimal*" (Emslie, Rush et al., 1997: 1033). There is no mention in the paper about any children attempting suicide. However, in the FDA's "Medical Review of Prozac," written in 2001 but not made public until 2003, there is a discussion about two children on Prozac attempting suicide (Center for Drug Evaluation and Research, 2001; Leo, 2004). Thus, between 1997 and 2003, doctors reading the published paper and trying to decide if Prozac should be used in children were not given all the information. Even by 2003, only those doctors who regularly peruse the FDA web site would have known about the two suicide attempts in the group of 48 Prozac-treated patients.

Under government pressure, the drug companies have released their unpublished data, while NIMH has still not explained the discrepancy between its own published and unpublished versions of the first Prozac for children paper. Also unclear are the details of how the data from this NIMH study became part of Eli Lilly's package that was submitted to the FDA for the evaluation of whether or not Prozac should be used in children. There is nothing wrong with Lilly simply using data in the public realm, but the data Lilly submitted to the FDA went beyond what was in the public realm *i.e.*, the two attempted suicides. Eli Lilly's access to NIMH's unpublished data suggests a close relationship between NIMH and the drug companies. The obvious question is: Did Lilly pay NIMH or the researchers for data that was the product of a taxpayer funded research project? Regardless of the monetary details surrounding the first Prozac study, by the time the second Prozac study was published in 2002, Emslie and his co-authors were either Lilly employees or paid consultants. And now, as of 2004, Emslie is still receiving money from NIMH to continue investigating these medicines in children.

When an investigator is simultaneously receiving funds from a non-profit institution and a for-profit company – one organization primarily committed to finding the truth, and one organization primarily committed to satisfying shareholders – it has to be extremely difficult to keep these allegiances straight. When a professor in this situation, at a scientific symposium for instance, claims that *"Studies show . . ."* is the professor referring to the published studies, or all the studies? As we are seeing, this qualifier has now become one of the essential pieces of information that goes into evaluating a scientific claim.

What is clear, though, is that, in general, all these studies are designed to give the drug the best chance of coming out ahead. For instance, the two Prozac studies, and several of the others, included a placebo washout phase, which involved putting all the patients on a placebo for a specified time period and then dropping those patients that got better. In the first Prozac study ten children were dropped from the study during the placebo washout.

The second Prozac study also had a unique twist, which consisted of a run-in phase to pre-select for drug responders (Emslie, et al., 2002; Dubitsky, 2004). All the Prozac-treated children in this study were given ten mg for the first week and children who did not respond, or who had negative responses, could then be dropped from the study. At the start of week two, the dose was increased to 20 mg. The subsequent statistical analysis only used children who had had at least one week of treatment with 20 mg. Thus, before the study even started, there was a mechanism in place to maximize any difference between the drug and placebo groups – the placebo group was pre-selected for *non-responders,* while the drug group was pre-selected for *responders.* Yet even with this advantage, for the prospectively defined primary outcome measure, 65 percent of the children on Prozac had a beneficial response compared to 53 percent of the placebo patients, a result that was not statistically significant. It was only by looking at other measures that clinical significance was found; on the patient- and parent-rated scales there was no advantage to Prozac, but on one of the clinician-rated scales there was a slight advantage to Prozac. Although Russell Katz of the FDA wrote, *"one could argue that this post hoc choice of primary outcome is inappropriate,"* the FDA accepted the post hoc change and approved Prozac for children in January 2003 (Center for Drug Evaluation and Research, 2002: 13). It was the only antidepressant that the FDA ever approved for use in childhood depression.

In 2003, when the British MHRA banned the use of these medications in children and teens, Prozac was spared. Not because the suicide profile was noticeably different, but because Prozac appears to offer more benefit than its competitors. Yet, according to the data, the efficacy of Prozac is not very significant. Using the researchers own criteria for defining an "improvement," and taking into account the large placebo effect, for every ten children it is given to, it maybe helps one patient.

Paxil (Paroxetine)

The course of child psychiatry was changed forever in 2001 when *The Journal of the American Academy of Child and Adolescent Psychiatry* published a study, which found that Paxil was appropriate for the treatment of emotional distress in children. The paper, authored by leaders in the child psychiatry profession, concluded that, *"Paroxetine is generally well tolerated and effective for major depression in adolescents"* (Keller et al., 2001: 762). At first, this paper seemed to justify the prescribing patterns of the past several years.

But, at the time the paper was published, it was clear to some people that there were major problems with the study (Jureidini and Tonkin, 2003). First, the study provided little evidence that Paxil was better than placebo. For the primary endpoint, the difference between the Paxil-treated and placebo groups was not significant (Laughren, 2004). Secondly, there were significant side effects in the Paxil-exposed children compared to those in the placebo group.

While the authors of the study vigorously defended their paper against the critics, the truth came out when internal, confidential company documents surfaced, supporting the critics instead of the company's own paid experts. The memo, written in October 1998 and stamped, *"For Internal Use Only,"* was a summary of the same Paxil study. It acknowledged that the study, at that point referred to as *Protocol 329*, had not demonstrated efficacy for Paxil and that "it would be commercially unacceptable to include a statement that efficacy had not been demonstrated, as this would undermine the profile of paroxetine" (GlaxoSmithKline, 1998).

In the published account of *Protocol 329*, the authors included an extensive list of 32 side effects such as nausea, vomiting, chest pain, etc. Although, ever since the SSRIs were approved for adults, there has been the suspicion that they lead to increased thoughts of suicide (Healy, 2003b), there is no mention of any children having any suicidal thoughts or attempting suicide in the published version of *Protocol 329*. Interestingly, six of the children on Paxil had *"emotional lability."*

The classification of some children with emotional lability was the proverbial straw that broke the camel's back: in reality, some of these "emotionally labile" children actually had suicidal thoughts (Healy 2004). At the urging of the British government, GlaxoSmithKline acknowledged that in *Protocol 329's* Paxil-treated group, there were 5 children out of 93 who had suicidal thoughts; in the placebo group none of the 89 children had suicidal thoughts. Prior to this revelation the average physician would have been left completely ignorant of this vital statistic.

The investigative news show *Prime Time Live* recently broadcast a segment about GlaxoSmithKline distributing a memo (different than the one mentioned above) to its sales force touting Paxil's, "remarkable efficacy and safety in the treatment of adolescent depression" in 2001, at a time when the company was fully aware that there were problems with Paxil (ABC, 2004). But far more problematic for the medical community, than a sales force being given a slanted view from sales managers is that doctors were given the same slanted view in medical journals from scientists. If the company is at fault for concealing data from its sales force, then what about the scientists who did the very same thing in the published paper? Whether you believe it was the pharmaceutical salespeople or the medical school professors who convinced clinicians to use these medicines, probably says a lot about your views of medicine in general. Shouldn't the media's focus really be on the journals, not the marketing memos? While the company's behaviour in the *Protocol 329* affair will probably be addressed via court proceedings, what about the behaviour of the scientists who are listed as authors of the published paper?

It would be interesting to know the time line of events, and the nature of the scientists' involvement with the Paxil study. For instance, at what point did the stated authors of the Paxil study even become involved with the project? Were they involved by 1998, when the company memo acknowledging the problems with the study was written, or did they join the project after the actual data was collected? If they were involved by 1998, and were aware of the results, then how do they defend their involvement in a paper whose stated "target" was "to effectively manage the dissemination of these data in order to minimize any potential negative impact"? When they published their paper, were they aware of negative data that GlaxoSmithKline was withholding about Paxil? As it stands now, the role the authors of the published paper played in all this is unclear. Much of this affair has still not come to light, but, because many of these scientists continue to make regular press appearances, they have ample chances to explain the parts they played in this matter.

Zoloft (Sertraline)

At the end of 1996, Pfizer submitted a request to the FDA for the approval of Zoloft as a treatment for Obsessive Compulsive Disorder (OCD) in children, and in October 1997 the FDA approved the request (Center for

Drug Evaluation and Research, 1997). Anyone reading the published literature on the use of Zoloft in children at that time would have learned of one suicidal act in a Zoloft-treated child in Pfizer's studies. Yet in the FDA's evaluation of the data up to that point, there were six instances of suicidal acts in children taking Zoloft (Center for Drug Evaluation and Research, 1997; Pfizer, 1997; Healy, 2004). Why the discrepancy between the published and unpublished data? The explanations are interesting. In one paper by Alderman and his colleagues, the authors decided to only publish side effects that occurred in ten percent or more of the patients, which excused them from reporting the fact that nine percent of the children on Zoloft in their study had engaged in a suicidal act (Alderman et al., 1998, cited in Healy, 2003).

In August of 2003, a major paper was published in *The Journal of the American Medical Association*, stating that Zoloft *"is an effective and well-tolerated short-term treatment for children and adolescents with Major Depressive Disorder"* (Wagner et al., 2003: 1033). For this paper, the authors combined the results of two smaller studies and collectively presented the findings (Wagner et al., 2003). Karen Wagner, the lead author, was also an author of some of the Paxil and Prozac studies in children.

It might seem odd that a company-sponsored paper would combine two studies into one paper. Publishing two positive papers would certainly seem to make a stronger case for the drug. After all, the headline, *"Two Studies Show . . .,"* or better yet, *"Multiple Studies Show . . ."* sounds much more convincing than *"One Study Has Shown . . ."* So why did the authors combine the two studies? It likely had something to do with the fact that, as stand-alone studies, one was a failure and one showed only a trend. Only by combining the two studies as one could statistical significance be reached.

Just as in the studies with Paxil and Prozac, doctors trying to weigh the pros and cons of prescribing these drugs were not given all the information in the medical literature; only by reading government reports (Committee on Safety of Medicines, 2004) would doctors have known that, individually, each trial was a failure. The headline could just as easily have been, *"Two Studies show that Zoloft Should Not Be Used in Children."*

Even by combining the two studies, of the children in the Zoloft group, 69 percent had a successful response, whereas 59 percent of the children in the placebo group experienced a successful response: not a large difference, but enough to make the headlines. Clearly, the marketing department, with plenty of help, was successful in its management of the negative information surrounding this study.

There is also an interesting nuance to their experimental design. The authors do not mention how many of the patients in this study had a history of psychiatric medication, but from their discussion, probably most of the patients had a history of SSRI treatment. One of the exclusion criteria for entry into this study was a *"history of failure to respond to a clinically adequate dosing regiment of an SSRI.*" In other words, those who have not responded to prior SSRI treatment were excluded, but it seems that another way to word this would be: *"Our study, designed to determine if SSRI treatment successfully treats depression,* will only use those children *who have been successfully treated with an SSRI for depression.*" In addition, 17 of the Zoloft-treated children, compared to 5 placebo-treated children, dropped out because of serious adverse events. This difference in adverse events between Zoloft and placebo groups was given little attention by the researchers, but did raise more attention at the FDA and in subsequent media articles.

According to the FDA report, in these two studies there were six suicide events in the Zoloft group and two in the placebo group. However, in the published paper it is not quite as clear. Regarding suicides, in one part of the paper the authors reported, *"the number of suicide attempts was the same in each treatment group, (2 for sertraline [Zoloft] and 2 for placebo)"* (Wagner et al, 2003: 1039). At least, this was the quote the press picked up on (Burton and Callahan, 2003). However, in another part of the paper, the authors also mention that in terms of suicidal ideation there were three events in the Zoloft group versus none in the placebo group. In addition, one Zoloft patient had an *"aggressive reaction."* This description of events did not make the press, or receive much attention from the authors, but it did receive attention from the regulators.

One defence of the paper's roundabout way of discussing the suicides might be that when the studies were being conducted, the suicide issue was not on the radar so it was overlooked. Only with the benefit of hindsight, once the issue of suicidality was raised, did a retrospective look at this study point to increased suicidality. The problem with this defence is that, by the time the Zoloft study was published, there were numerous hints about a link between the SSRIs and suicides in children. Even the authors acknowledge in the paper that regulators in the United States and United Kingdom are looking at the suicide issue (p. 1038), yet they still sidestep the suicide data in their own study.

It is surprising that the peer reviewers of the Zoloft study did not think to ask more questions about the study, such as: (1) Why not mention the findings of each study individually in the paper? (2) What about the discrepancy between the withdrawal rates of the Zoloft and placebo groups? (3) What about only a ten percent difference between the drug and placebo groups?

One of the investigators involved with the Zoloft study, who was not an author and, apparently, not privy to drafts of the paper, eventually wrote a letter to *JAMA*, after the study was published, pointing out some of the very concerns that the reviewers should have spotted. Though the letter unfortunately went unpublished, it stated that the conclusions of the paper should have been: *"Sertraline is ineffective when compared to placebo and is associated with increased adverse events"* (Garland, 2004).

The American College of Neuropsychopharmacology's Response

As the child psychiatry profession was in the midst of a public relations problem, the American College of Neuropsychopharmacology published their *Preliminary Report of the Task Force on Suicidal Behavior in Youth*. The task force members claimed that, *"there is sufficient evidence to conclude that, overall, SSRIs are effective in treating depression in children and adolescents"* (American College of Neuropsychopharmacology, 2004: 4). The task force was composed of ten members who were pivotal in the medical community's acceptance of treating young children with these drugs. Three of the members, Graham Emslie, Karen Wagner, and Neal Ryan, were authors of the Prozac, Zoloft, and Paxil studies mentioned above. In light of the fact that the papers these authors wrote are the source of all the confusion, it is difficult to know how to characterize their following statement, *"all data held by FDA or pharmaceutical companies should be made rapidly available to allow ACNP and other research organizations to conduct an independent evaluation of the risks and benefits of SSRIs"* (American College of Neuropsychopharmacology, 2004: 11). Their call for openness seems hollow when one considers the way the results from their own papers were reported.

The ANCP has declared that, based on their analysis of confidential data, there is no link between suicide and SSRIs; and while they cannot share all the data with the scientific community, because of their credentials, we should trust their analysis – conflicts of interest aside. Yet, this is not the way science functions.

Two Papers from the United Kingdom

In the spring of 2004, two papers, which brought worldwide attention to the issue, were published in British medical journals, not American journals. This turn of events was hardly surprising since at every step of the way the British medical community had shown more scepticism. The first paper, published in the April 2004 issue of *The British Medical Journal*, was a review of the SSRIs for children by Jon Jureidini and his colleagues (Jureidini et al., 2004). They concluded that the authors of the original papers had exaggerated the benefits and downplayed the risks. The paper, whose importance cannot be underestimated, received a tremendous amount of media coverage. Yet, Jureidini et al did not really uncover any new data, nor did they find some "smoking-gun" hidden away in a drug company basement. He and his co-authors summarized the data that the original authors had mentioned in their studies, and their message was clear: Before the use of these of these drugs becomes too entrenched, it is time to pause and take another look at the scientific evidence. Unlike the members of the mainstream press, who uncritically reported the scientists' conclusions without apparently looking at the data themselves, Jureidini and his colleagues looked at the actual data. For instance, the original authors of the Zoloft paper thought that a ten percent difference between the Zoloft and placebo group was significant, but as the Jureidini paper pointed out, or reminded people, this statistic is not very clinically significant. The problem for academic medicine is that when the entire issue is approached as a rational scientific enterprise, where the data drives the treatment decisions – rather than what appears to have been occurring where the decision to prescribe these drugs occurred well before the data was even published – then it is clear that there is little justification for the current prescribing patterns.

Two weeks later, *The Lancet* published a review by Whittington and colleagues that brought even more attention to the controversy (Whittington et al., 2004). These authors showed that once the unpublished literature is included in the risk-benefit analysis of these drugs, the benefits do not outweigh the risks. With the publication of the Jureidini and Whittington papers in mainstream medical journals, the SSRIs were in more trouble. The editorial in *The Lancet* following the Whittington paper could not have been clearer "*That such an event [suicide] could be precipitated by a supposedly beneficial drug is a catastrophe. The idea of that drug's use being based on selective reporting of favourable research should be unimaginable . . .*" (Editors, 2004: 1335).

What seems to bother *The Lancet* editors, and others, is that, as a body of research, there seems to be a systematic bias towards downplaying the suicide issue. Whether there is a link between suicide and the antidepressants, and whether there is significant benefit to the antidepressants are still valid scientific questions, which will eventually be answered. However, so far, the manner in which the academic community has handled the data calls into question who will now investigate theses issues. The next time one of these papers is published, the logical question on many people's minds will be: What about the *unpublished* studies?

Of course, the drug companies and authors of these studies will argue about the data mentioned in this paper (Clary, 2004) but, whatever the arguments, the data were incriminating enough to convince two governments to intercede; the Americans with a warning label, and the British with an outright ban on several of the medications for people under 18 years of age.

However, besides concerns about suicide, there is a very good reason for not taking the drugs: They simply don't work very well. In all these studies, the difference between the percentages of favourable responses in the drug-treated group compared to favourable responses in the placebo group is minimal (for a discussion of this issue in adults see Kirsch et al., 2002). In the risk-benefit analysis, given such little benefit, there is little justification for putting up with the suicide risk. If the studies had shown significant benefits, the suicide risk would have been better tolerated by the regulatory agencies.

Attention Deficit Disorder

Concerta and some Tricks of the Trade

In November 2004, while much of the press was focusing on the problems with the SSRIs, an interview was published, which highlighted the fact that questions about scientific credibility are not limited to the SSRI research, but apply to the whole field of child psychiatry (Hearn, 2004). The interview was with William Pelham, a prominent ADHD researcher, who has served as a voice of moderation in the debate about behavioural versus pharmacological therapy. In his interview he provides fascinating insight into the case of how evidence-based medicine was manufactured for a relatively new drug called Concerta, a slow-release version of methylphenidate (Ritalin). On the web page of the ALZA Corporation, a subsidiary of McNeil Pharmaceuticals (*Concerta.net*), there are statements extolling the benefits of Concerta: one being that 96 percent of the children taking the drug do not experience significant side effects (appetite, growth and sleep). Pelham's study is one of three studies cited as supporting evidence for this claim (Pelham et al., 2001). However, in his interview, Pelham points out how misleading this statement is, because his study started with children who had already been taking Concerta and who had experienced no significant side effects—children who exhibited side effects would not have gotten in the study to begin with. Pelham is even surprised that the FDA allows ALZA to use his study to make the claims it does. In addition, Pelham mentions that the company pressured him to delete a paragraph he wrote about the importance of behavioural therapy.

It gets even more interesting. Pelham discusses his experience in collaborating in a follow-up paper (Wilens et al., 2003), in which the company did the data analysis and coordinated the writing of the paper. In Pelham's words, *"I insisted on seeing the analyses and having major inputs into the manuscript, and it was like pulling teeth to get wording and analyses changed. It was like a whitewash – a praise to Concerta."* Even more problematic, Pelham reports that the *Journal of the American Academy of Child and Adolescent Psychiatry* sent back the paper for revisions twice, but that he was not involved with the revisions and never signed off on the paper – which was eventually published anyway.

But pharmaceutical company tricks aside, here is the problem for the academic community: Pelham's co-authors are the leaders in the field of ADHD research and, because they have played a major role in convincing the American medical community to use these medications, the obvious question becomes, *"What was their involvement with the study?"* Is it true, as Pelham has implied that the companies were in charge, and the researchers essentially just added their names to the study? Not only are they the leaders in the field, they are also on record as declaring themselves the sole arbiters of scientific truth. In their International Consensus Statement (Barkley, Cook et al., 2002), they compare those who question the widespread use of stimulant medication in children to members of the Flat Earth Society, and they state: *"ADHD should be depicted in the media as realistically and accurately as it is depicted in science."* In an ironic twist, it now seems that if the media wants to aim for the bar these scientists have set they should aim low, rather than high. The problem for those who wrote this statement is that the media finally appears to have caught up with such obvious deficiencies in how the *science* was conducted. The predicament for the mainstream medical journals is that it is the members of the media – and not peer reviewers and journal editors – who are picking up on the deficiencies in this research. In fact, many experts who pointed out these deficiencies (Breggin, 1999; Breggin, 2000) were routinely ignored by the mainstream journals.

ADHD Neuroimaging Research

Besides clinical research, basic science research also has clear institutional biases when it comes to investigating medication side effects. An illustration of this fact is evident in the ADHD neuroimaging research. For anyone familiar with the scientific method there would seem to be three logical choices for groups of children to examine in imaging research: unmedicated ADHD children, medicated ADHD children, and controls. A simple experiment using these three groups would seem to answer many questions. With three groups of children in each experiment there are multiple possibilities for comparisons. For instance a comparison between the medicated and unmedicated ADHD children could answer questions about the effect of medications on brain development. This type of comparison is often done between controls and users of illicit drugs, with any anatomical difference being attributed to the effect of a drug. Another comparison, between unmedicated ADHD children and controls, could provide insight into the "biological" basis for ADHD, yet even with this comparison any anatomical difference might be due to environmental stressors.

The most problematic comparison, in terms of interpretation, would be between medicated ADHD children and controls, because any anatomical differences could be due to a medication effect, an organic deficit, or some combination of the two. Yet, for 30 years, and in over 30 studies, this comparison has been a mainstay of ADHD imaging researchers. Baughman has pointed this out for many years (1998); yet, for the most part, the ADHD researchers have ignored this confounding variable and declared that their results show a biological basis of ADHD, although one could just as easily interpret their results as confirmation that stimulant medication is harmful to the developing brain.

In the past few years, the ADHD-imaging researchers have finally acknowledged that prior medication use in the subjects is a confounding variable, and they have started to use non-medicated ADHD children in their studies. While this would seem to simplify their studies, somehow, it has made them more complicated. A comparison between two recent studies, both funded by NIMH, is illuminating. One study, with the first author being Xavier Castellanos, was published in 2002. The second study, with the first author being Elizabeth Sowell, was published in 2003. Both studies had three groups of children: medicated ADHD children, unmedicated ADHD children, and controls. Yet only the Castellanos study reported results about the comparison between the unmedicated ADHD children and medicated ADHD children – results which could make a case for prescribing or not prescribing stimulants. A major finding of the study, according to the authors and the corresponding NIMH press release (NIMH, 2002), was that the researchers found no neuro-anatomical differences between the unmedicated ADHD and medicated ADHD children, thus the conclusion that stimulants are not harmful to the developing brain. Probably never in the history of drug research has a drug been given such a clean bill of health by a government agency based on such limited data – a single study. Especially since the study also failed to provide any details about the specifics of medication history, such as: what medications the children were taking; information about dosages they had been given; or for how many years the children had been medicated. Apparently the specifics about medication history were not problematic for NIMH's interpretation (Leo and Cohen, 2003; Cohen and Leo, 2004).

But just a year later, all of a sudden, the specifics about medication history were problematic. Variable medication histories were now the very reason given by the Sowell team for *not* reporting on the comparison between medicated and unmedicated ADHD children – even more problematic, they cite Castellanos as support for not reporting the data. Is it possible that Sowell's team did the comparison and found evidence that stimulants are harmful, and then decided not to publish the data? At this point no one knows, but if so, the results would certainly run counter to NIMH's message (and academic psychiatry in general) that children diagnosed with ADHD should be medicated. The suspicion seems justified when one considers that, for 30 years, prior medication use in ADHD subjects never got in the way of ADHD researchers attributing their findings to an organic pathology. Even in the Sowell study, medication history is not a problem when it comes to comparing medicated ADHD children to controls. Certainly, most ADHD researchers must be interested in Sowell's omitted comparison between the medicated and unmedicated ADHD children. In the Castellanos study, the comparison was worthy of a NIMH press release, yet for the same comparison in the Sowell study no one is curious about the comparison? The Sowell researchers have refused to release any data about the comparison between medicated and unmedicated children, and NIMH has denied a Freedom of

Information Act Request to see the data, even though, according to NIH's web page, there is no question that researchers should be sharing data. In their words "*There are many reasons to share data from NIH-supported studies. Sharing data reinforces open scientific inquiry, encourages diversity of analysis and opinion, promotes new research, makes possible the testing of new or alternative hypotheses and methods of analysis, supports studies on data collection methods and measurement, facilitates the education of new researchers, enables the exploration of topics not envisioned by the initial investigators, and permits the creation of new data when data from multiple sources are combined*" (NIH, 2002).

Is someone at NIH, or NIMH, supposed to enforce these guidelines? While the paragraph makes a great case for sharing data, evidently, the words are meaningless. NIH can say all it wants about the need to share data but, in the case of the Sowell data, NIH's actions – more like a for-profit company – are completely at odds with their published views. In one sense, since the FDA hearings on these issues, the pharmaceutical companies have been more forthcoming with data than NIMH.

What Are Clinicians Supposed to Think?

The problem for academic medicine is that the average doctor, who wants to make an evidenced-based decision about the use of a certain treatment, should be able to turn to experiments published in the medical literature for guidance. Unfortunately, in the case of using psychotropic drugs in children, this is not possible.

A major lesson to be learned from the past decade is the importance of reading the primary literature, because as soon as the primary literature is published it gets twisted or "*spun*" into a marketing message. Of course that will happen in marketing brochures, but it is also true for book chapters, professional talks, and review articles. A classic example of this trend relates to an article in *JAMA* that examined the efficacy of St. John's Wort for the treatment of depression (Hypericum Depression Trial Study Group, 2002). Besides establishing a St. John's Wort group and a placebo group, the study also included a group of patients who were treated with Zoloft. And, although both St. John's Wort and Zoloft failed to beat the placebo, the paper and subsequent news coverage focused primarily on the failure of St. John's Wort. In the words of the authors, "*On the two primary outcome measures, neither sertraline nor Hypericum [St. John's Wort] was significantly different from placebo*" (Hypericum Depression Trial Study Group, 2002: 1807). In a sign of the times, at the end of the paper, the authors' affiliations were listed. It is hard to know what to make of the fact that just about every drug company in existence is listed; if you are concerned about conflicts of interest, it is shocking.

Putting the authors' conflicts aside, because even with the conflicts their findings could be correct, more problematic is the *JAMA* editors' choice of two outside experts to summarize and explain the findings. With the entire worldwide medical community to choose from, somehow, the two invited experts also happened to have worked for Pfizer at one point: one as a consultant, and one as a management scientist (Kupfer and Frank, 2002). Can anyone really be surprised that their accompanying commentary found little fault with Zoloft but numerous problems with St. John's Wort (See Sharav, 2002 for a discussion of this issue and other conflicts of interest)?

Many people want to blame the FDA for the approval of antidepressant use in children, or for not withdrawing the drugs from the market sooner, but out of seven requests from pharmaceutical companies for FDA approval, the FDA rejected six drugs, the only antidepressant they approved for children was for Prozac. But, while the FDA rejected six studies, the rest of the medical community accepted them. Doctors accepted these drugs and prescribed them so willingly not because they were given free pens, free dinners, or even free trips (Mizik and Jacobson, In press). They put their trust in the drugs because they were backed by papers which were: written by professors at the major academic medical centres; approved by peer reviewers; published in the major medical journals; cited in review articles; discussed at meetings; defended by The American College of Neuropsychopharmacology; and, underlying everything, given NIMH's stamp of approval (National Institute of Mental Health, 2001). In short, these papers were the talk of the town. You can hardly fault the average physician for putting faith in them.

Another way of looking at this entire affair is that the FDA had to actively intercede only because of a systemic problem in academic medicine. The FDA did not just have to deal with the problematic side effect of a medication; it had to deal with a profession in denial. If academic medicine had been working correctly, the FDA's drastic step would not have been necessary. Not only has the psychiatric profession fought the FDA every step of the way – for the most part, it has still not acknowledged the problem (Koplewicz, 2004). Many of the SSRI defenders point out that in the clinical trials none of the children with suicidal thoughts actually committed suicide. However, it seems counterintuitive for these defenders to downplay the relevance of suicidal thoughts, when it is the presence of suicidal thoughts that supposedly justified writing the prescriptions in the first place.

It is hard to dissect these studies and know where to draw the line between "science" and "marketing." There are many proposals for solutions to the problem, some of which have been written about by others, some of which are already in place now, and some of which will soon be implemented, but the single best way to prevent this from happening again is for doctors to pay more attention to the primary literature, and to place less reliance on second-hand sources. By now, virtually everyone involved in medicine is aware of the need to take a healthy dose of scepticism before reading pharmaceutical company brochures or when attending talks by pharmaceutical representatives. It is now evident that those doses of scepticism need to be taken, or maybe even increased, when reading medical journals.

At the end of 2004, the MHRA issued the somewhat surprising statement that people suffering from minor depression should *not* be given antidepressant medications (MHRA), something which critics have been saying for years. Needless to say, another way of looking at their acknowledgement is that it was a confession, of sorts, that the medical community has inappropriately treated thousands of people with these medications, and that, instead of antidepressants, people with minor depression should have been treated with talk therapy. Overnight, a major medical institution essentially took a giant step back from the disease model of mental illness and from ten years of psychiatry research claiming that mild depression results from a biological deficit due to faulty genes (of course, definitions of "minor depression" will certainly vary from one doctor to another or from one committee to another). Considering that the placebo response was so high in studies of antidepressant use in children – just seeing a doctor helped many of these children improve – it is quite possible that many of the children in these studies suffered from minor depression and never needed antidepressants in the first place, at least according to the MHRA's new guidelines.

For a moment, let's leave out all talk of numbers, statistics, percentages, rating scales, and placebos; let's put aside all the speculations about genetic predispositions and unproven theories about serotonin; and let's simply allow for a dose of common sense to enter the discussion. Of course children suffer, and they often need help, however, during the past decade the widespread acceptance by the medical community of the idea that childhood distress is a "disease" in need of medication, evidently, had more to do with marketing than science.

References

ABC (2004). Drug maker withheld paxil safety data. *Prime Time Live* December 9, 2004. Available: http://abcnews.go.com/Health/print?id=311956.

Alderman, J., R. Wolkow, et al. (1998). Sertraline treatment of children and adolescents with obsessive-compulsive disorder or depression: Pharmacokinetics, tolerability, and efficacy. *Journal of Child and Adolescent Psychiatry* 37, 386-394.

American College of Neuropsychopharmacology (2004). Executive summary: Preliminary report of the task force on SSRIs and suicidal behavior in youth. Available: http://www.acnp.org/exec_summary.pdf.

Barkley, R., E. Cook, et al. (2002). International consensus statement on ADHD. *Clinical Child and Family Psychology Review* 5, 89-111.

Breggin, P. (1999). Psychostimulants in the treatment of children diagnosed with ADHD: Part II – Adverse effects on brain and behavior. *Ethical Human Sciences and Services* 1, 213-241.

Breggin, P. (2000). A Critical Analysis of the NIMH Multimodal Treatment Study for Attention-Deficit Hyperactivity Disorder. *Ethical Human Sciences and Services* 2, 63-72.

Burton, T. and P. Callahan (2003). Antidepressant use for kids gains support, August 27, 2003. *Wall Street Journal*. Available: <http://www.healthyplace.com/Communities/Depression/treatment/antidepressants/articles/014.asp.

Castellanos, F. X., P. P. Lee, et al. (2002). Developmental trajectories of brain volume abnormalities in children and adolescents with attention-deficit hyperactivity disorder. *Journal of the American Medical Association* 288, 1740-1748.

Center for Drug Evaluation and Research (1997). Approval package for NDA 1938/S-017 and S-018: Medical review of sertraline hydrochloride. Available: http://www.fda.gov/cder/foi/nda/97/019839ap.pdf.

Center for Drug Evaluation and Research (2001). Application 18-936-SE-064. Medical review of fluoxetine, July 2001. Available: http://www.fda.gov/cder/foi/nda/2003/18936S064_Prozac%20Pulvules_medr.pdf.

Center for Drug Evaluation and Research (2002). Application number 18-936/SE5-064, Administrative Documents for fluoxetine. Available: http://www.fda.gov/cder/foi/nda/2003/18936S064_Prozac%20Pulvules_admindocs.pdf.

Clary, C.M. (2004). Sertraline pediatric depression trial met highest standards of study design and reporting. *British Medical Journal* 329, 879.

Cohen, D. and J.T. Leo (2004). An update on ADHD neuroimaging research. *The Journal of Mind and Behavior* 25, 161-166.

Committee on Safety of Medicines (2004). Selective serotonin reuptake inhibitors (SSRIs) – overview of regulatory status and CSM advice relating to major depressive disorder (MDD) in children and adolescents: Summary of clinical trials. Available:

http://medicines.mhra.gov.uk/ourwork/monitorsafequalmed/safetymessages/ssrioverviewclintrialdata_101203.htm.

Dubitsky, C. (2004). Review and evaluation of clinical data placebo-controlled antidepressant studies in pediatric patients, FDA. Available: http://www.fda.gov/ohrms/dockets/ac/04/briefing/2004-4065b1-08-TAB06-Dubitsky-Review.pdf>.

Editors (2004). Depressing research. *The Lancet* 363, 1335..

Emslie, G.J., J. Heiligenstein, et al. (2002). Fluoxetine for acute treatment of depression in children and adolescents: A placebo-controlled, randomized clinical trial. *Journal of American Academy of Child and Adolescent Psychiatry* 41, 1205-1215.

Emslie, G.J., A.J. Rush, et al. (1997). A double-blind, randomized, placebo-controlled trial of fluoxetine in children and adolescents with depression. *Archives of General Psychiatry* 54, 1031-1037.

Garland, J. (2004). Letter to Editor, *Journal of the American Medical Association*, (unpublished). Available: http://www/ahrp.org/infomail/04/01/09.html.

GlaxoSmithKline (1998). Seraxat/Paxil adolescent depression: Position piece on the phase III clinical studies, Executive summary. Available: http://ahrp.org/risks/SSRI0204/GSKpaxil/index.html.

Grinfeld, J. (1998). Psychoactive Medications and Kids: New Initiatives Launched. *Psychiatric Times* 69.

Healy, D. (2003a). *Let Them Eat Prozac*. Toronto, James Lorimer & Company.

Healy, D. (2003b). Lines of evidence on the risks of suicide with selective serotonin reuptake inhibitors. *Psychotherapy and Psychosomatics* 72, 71-79.

Healy, D. (2004). Suicidal evidence not addressed by FDA: Letter from David Healy to Peter J. Pitts, Associate Commissioner for external relations, Food and Drug Administration (unpublished). Available: http://ahrp.org/risks/healy/fda0204.html.

Hearn, K. (2004). Here, kiddie, kiddie. *AlterNet.com*. Available: http://www.alternet.org/drugreporter/20594/.

Hypericum Depression Trial Study Group (2002). Effect of hypericum perforatum (St John's Wort) in major depressive disorder. *Journal of the American Medical Association* 287, 1807-1814.

Jureidini, J.N., C.J. Doecke, et al. (2004). Efficacy and safety of antidepressants for children and adolescents. *British Medical Journal* 328, 879-883.

Jureidini, J.N. and A.L. Tonkin (2003). Paroxetine in major depression. *Journal of American Academy of Child and Adolescent Psychiatry* 42, 514.

Keller, M.B., N.D. Ryan, et al. (2001). Efficacy of paroxetine in the treatment of adolescent major depression: A randomized, controlled trial. *Journal of American Academy of Child and Adolescent Psychiatry* 40, 762-772.

Kirsch, I., T.J. Moore, et al. (2002). The Emperor's new drugs: An analysis of antidepressant medication data submitted to the US Food and Drug Administration. *Prevention and Treatment*. Available: http://www.journals.apa.org/prevention/volume5/pre0050023a.html.

Koplewicz, H. (1997). *It's Nobody's Fault: New Hope and Help for Difficult Children and Their Parents*, Three Rivers Press.

Koplewicz, H. (2004). Misguided resistance to appropriate treatment for adolescent depression. *Journal of Child and Adolescent Psychopharmacology* 14, 7.

Kupfer, D. and E. Frank (2002). Placebo in clinical trials for depression. *Journal of the American Medical Association* 287, 1853-1854.

Laughren, T.P. (2004). January 5, 2004 FDA Memorandum; Background comments for February 2, 2004 meeting of the Psychopharmacological drugs advisory committee (PDAC) and pediatric subcommittee of the anti-infective drugs advisory committee. Available: **http://www.fda.gov/ohrms/dockets/ac/04/briefing/2004-4065b1-04-Tab02-Laughren-Jan5.pdf**.

Leo, J. (2004). NIMH guilty too? *Psychiatric News* 39, 31.

Leo, J. and D. Cohen (2003). Broken brains or flawed studies? A critical review of ADHD neuroimaging studies. *The Journal of Mind and Behavior* 24, 29-56.

MHRA (2004). Safey of selective serotonin reuptake inhibitors. Available: **http://www.mhra.gov.uk/news/2004/SSRI_Letter_061204.pdf**.

Mizik, N. and R. Jacobson (In press). Are physicians "Easy Marks'?" Quantifying the effects of detailing and sampling on new prescriptions. *Management Science*.

Mosholder, A.D. (2004). Executive summary, Suicidality in pediatric clinical trials with paroxetine and other antidepressant drugs: Follow up to 9-4-03 consult. Availabe: **http://psychrights.org/Research/Digest/AntiDepressants/Mosholder/MosholderReport.pdf**.

National Institute of Mental Health (2001). Let's talk about depression, NIH publication 01-4162. Available: **http://www.nimh.nih.gov/publicat/letstalk.cfm**.

NIH (2002). NIH announces draft statement on sharing research data. *Notice: NOT-OD-02-035*. Available: **http://www.niams.nih.gov/rtac/funding/grants/notice/notod02-035.htm**.

NIMH (2002). Brain shrinkage in ADHD not caused by medications, **http://www.nimh.nih.gov/events/pradhdmri.cfm**.

Pelham, W., E.M. Gnagy, et al. (2001). Once-a-day concerta methylphenidate versus three-times-daily methylphenidate in laboratory and natural settings. *Pediatrics* 107, E105.

Pfizer (1997). Expert report on the clinical documentation of sertraline hydrochloride for obsessive compulsive disorder in pediatric patients. Available: **http://www.healyprozac.com/GhostlyData/expertreport.htm**.

Sharav, V. (2002). Conflicts of interest in clinical trials. *Presentation before U.S. army Medical Department and the Henry M. Jackson foundation for the advancement of military medicine*. Available: **http://ahrp.org/testimonypresentations/armymeddept.php**.

Sowell, E.R., Thompson, P.M. et al. (2003). Cortical abnormalities in children and adolescents with attention-deficit hyperactivity disorder. *The Lancet* 362, 1699-1707.

Wagner, K.D., P. Ambrosini, et al. (2003). Efficacy of sertaline in the treatment of children and adolescents with major depressive disorder: Two randomized controlled trials. *Journal of the American Medical Association* 290, 1033-1093.

Whittington, C.J., T. Kendall, et al. (2004). Selective serotonin reuptake inhibitors in childhood depression: Systematic review of published versus unpublished data. *The Lancet* 363, 1341-1345.

Wilens, T.E., W. Pelham, et al. (2003). ADHD treatment with once-daily OROS methylphenidate: Interim 12-month results from a long-term open-label study. *Journal of American Academy of Child and Adolescent Psychiatry* 42, 424-433.

7
Adolescent in-patient units: Changing the therapeutic philosophy

Sami Timimi · Elisse Moody

Introduction

Our understanding of the 'institutional' child has changed. This article tries to track some of the key factors influencing Western societies changing visions and practices in relation to children deemed unfit or unable to continue living with their families because of deviance in their behaviour, thoughts and/or feelings. In particular we concentrate on the historical context that led, first to the birth, and then to the growth of psychiatric in-patient institutions for children and adolescents.

In the second part of this chapter we describe our experience in changing the therapeutic culture at an adolescent in-patient unit in the United Kingdom (Ash Villa) from a more medical model dominated organizing framework to a more psychosocial one. We describe the constraining factors militating against such a change and how we attempted to overcome these.

Historical context

The immaturity of children is a biological fact of life. The ways in which this immaturity is understood and made meaningful is a fact of culture (La Fontaine, 1979, Prout and James, 1997). Viewed through a historical lens we can see that each historical period has created a novel version of the child. The developing images of childhood are not simply abandoned over time instead fragments from each period are incorporated into the succeeding period's ideas of childhood (Hendrick, 1997). Concepts of childhood, normality, deviance and child rearing practices are neither timeless nor universal but instead rooted in the past and reshaped in the present.

The same can be said for concepts of mental distress/illness, which change vertically over time as well as being different horizontally, in other words between different cultures. The discipline of psychiatry took shape in European asylums. According to Foucault, the emergence of large institutions in which "unreasonable" people were housed was not a progressive medical venture but an act of social exclusion (Foucault, 1971).

Psychiatry was the direct product of this act, with the rise of psychiatry being more the consequence than the cause of the rise of the insane asylum. Psychiatry only began to flourish once large numbers of inmates were crowded into asylums (Porter, 1987). A broader understanding of the role of adolescent in-patient units thus requires us to examine the broader historical/cultural dynamics within which these first came into existence and then changed. It requires us to examine the history of the institutionalized child in the West.

Psychiatrists first came to deal with children during the era of the large asylums of the nineteenth century where children were occasionally admitted alongside adults. Physicians favoured removal of some children from their homes to establish control unhindered by parental and family interference (Parry-Jones, 1990). However, at this point in history child and adolescent psychiatry as a discipline had not been established and it was rare for problematic behaviour in children to be viewed through a medical/psychological lens.

In late nineteenth century Europe and North America something of a perceived crises was occurring in the social structures of the time and children were often at the heart of the resulting political debates. Prior to the nineteenth century there were few voices raised against child labour. For most children, labouring was held to be a condition that would teach them numeracy, economics, social and moral principles (Hendrick, 1997). This view would soon be challenged. During the course of the nineteenth century a new construction of childhood was being put together where the wage-earning child would no longer be considered to be the norm. Instead childhood would soon be seen as constituting a separate and distinct life stage that required protection and fostering through school education. There are several explanations for this fundamental change. The scale and intensity of exploitation of children appalled many and the scale and intensity of the industrialization process itself equally appalled these critics. The plight of the factory child became symbolic of the profound and confusing changes that were occurring in Western society. The campaigners for reform had their roots in eighteenth century psychological, educational and philosophical developments and wished to promote a childhood that they considered more suitable for a civilized and Christian nation. With the growth of the first mass working class political movements that were also complaining about the brutalization and dehumanization of their children, the middle and upper classes became concerned about unstable social conditions and issues relating to public order became matters of national security (Rothman, 1984, Davidoff and Hall, 1987, and Pearson, 1983).

As the century moved on, the growing economic success of industrial capitalism resulted in a growing demand for a semi-skilled, skilled and educated work force, lessening the economic need for child labour and increasing the demand for education (Zelizer, 1998). Many reformers also associated child labour with slavery and looked to the anti-slavery movement of the period to draw analogies (Cunningham, 1991). The effect of the comparison of child wage earners to slaves furthered the view that their condition rendered them un-free. There was also a fear that the natural order of parents, and particularly fathers in supporting their children, was being inverted through the demand for child labour in factories at the expense of adult males. This led to a fear in the ruling classes that the neglect of children could easily lead, not only to damnation of souls, but also to a social revolution (Cunningham, 1991, Pearson, 1983). The growing influence of the campaigners coupled with the fears of the ruling classes thus led to the first piece of effective legislation in 1833 in the United Kingdom, which prohibited selective employment of children under nine and limited the working day to eight hours for those aged between nine and thirteen (Cunningham, 1995). Although initially making little difference in practice, the ideal situation had been formulated and posed and for the rest of the century, reformers, educationalists, politicians and social scientists strove to make real the ideal through two further reconstructions- the reformed juvenile delinquent and the compulsorily schooled child.

By the mid nineteenth century many of the middle class reformers were using a concept of childhood that was at odds with what they saw as the childhood of the poor and the neglected. Their intention was to make these children conform to a middle class notion of a properly constituted childhood, characterized by a state of dependence (Pearson, 1983). Where poor parents failed to rear such a child it was determined that parental discipline for delinquents should be provided by reformatory schools (Carpenter, 1853, Pearson, 1983, Pinchbeck and Hewitt, 1973). Young 'delinquents', and by implication all those other 'neglected' working class children, were exhibiting features which were the reverse of what the reformers desired to see in childhood. Thus, children had to be restored to the 'true' position of childhood (Manton, 1976). In order to understand the significance of these developments it has to be remembered that the movement to create a separate order of juvenile justice emerged from the debate on child labour, the economic and political upheavals of the nineteenth century and the increasing popularity of school as a means of class control (Hendrick, 1997).

Consequently, the writings of the reformers reflects their convictions about the nature of social order at a time when the middle classes were anxious about what it deemed was rebellious and aggressive attitudes and behaviour from those young people (and their parents) who frequented the streets of urban areas (May, 1973). The question facing politicians at that time was how to build a healthy, cooperative society with a cohesive social fabric to replace the perceived chaos and immorality of that time (Selleck, 1985, Pearson, 1983). A new conception of juvenile delinquency, and with it a new way of defining an ideal childhood was seen as part of the answer (May, 1973).

In their approach to reforming the juvenile delinquent many made the implicit assumption that in the long run only education would prevent the dangerous classes from continually reproducing their malevolent characteristics. The birth of the idea of 'willing obedience' through education was another step towards the coming of age of industrial democracy where the idea of 'rule by consent' was to become the norm (Pearson, 1983). For the reformers the idea of effective schooling now became paramount. The reconstruction of the factory child through the prism of dependency and ignorance was a necessary precursor to mass education in that it helped prepare opinion for shifts in the child's identity from wage earner to school pupil and for a reduction in the income of working class families that would result from the loss of the child's earning. It further paved the way for an important new development; that of introducing the state into the parent/child relationship. Not only had the reformers put aside the financial hardships many working class families would suffer as a result of the ending of the child labourer, but in addition they depicted the parents of such families as collaborators in the exploitation of their own children and so introduced a new way regulating family feeling too; if children were useful and produced money, they were not being properly loved (Zelizer, 1998).

The new school system threw aside the child's knowledge that was derived from their parents, community, peer group and personal experience and instead demanded a state of ignorance. It required upon the pain of punishment, usually physical, a form of behaviour accompanied by a set of related attitudes, which reinforced the child's dependence and vulnerability, and, in terms of deference towards established authorities, its social class (Humphries, 1981). The wage-earning child was no longer a proper child and therefore had to be made innocent of such adult behaviour. School also reinforced the idea of the child as being in need (for example of learning and of particular forms of discipline). It also further institutionalized the separation of children from society, confirming upon them a separate identity- their proper place now being in the classroom (Hendrick, 1992, 1997). When in the late nineteenth century the church and state began to enforce schooling, signs of opposition from parents began to surface in many Western countries. Much of this opposition was not to education itself, but to the syllabus, the system of controls and the fines given for non-attendance. At the same time enforced school attendance was seen by many children as depriving them of the opportunity of contributing to the family budget, a task many viewed with pride (Cunningham, 1995). However, by the dawn of the twentieth century the principle of compulsory education for all was well established in most Western nations.

It is within this historical/political context that 'institutional' responses to childhood problems of the time should be viewed. Thus many children, particularly those perceived to be a threat to the dominant order were 'contained' first in workhouses (or poor houses in North America) and then later in the nineteenth century in reformatory schools set up for detention, training and rehabilitation (Bridgeland, 1971). Borstals were then established in the UK in 1908 to train young offenders deemed to need higher levels of security than provided by reformatory schools (Barman, 1934). Thus much of the cultural response was via overt methods of social control through education/juvenile justice institutions that had a strong class character with the children of the working classes being perceived as the biggest threat to the existing social order. Psychiatrists had little to do with these populations.

By the late nineteenth century, partly under the impact of schooling and partly as a result of growing concern about poverty and its possible political consequences, a prolonged and unprecedented public discussion about the physical and mental condition of children began (Sutherland, 1984). One development above all others turned children into attractive research subjects, namely the opportunities afforded to investigators by mass schooling. School made children available to professionals like sociologists, psychologists and doctors, all of whom sought to do scientific surveys of pupils (Sutherland, 1984). Now children found themselves being examined under the influence of science. Mass schooling revealed the extent of mental and physical handicap amongst pupils which, together with a growing anxiety about racial degeneration and the effects of poverty, led a variety of professionals and middle class parents to become anxious about the quality of the child population leading to a great interest in the subject of human development (Wooldridge, 1995).

By the early twentieth century child welfare was achieving a new social and political identity, with a shift in emphasis toward maximizing children's potential (Baistow, 1995). This was thought politically, to be in the national interest. At that time in Western society policy was being developed that stressed the importance of national efficiency with an emphasis on education, racial hygiene, responsible parenthood, social purity and preventative medicine (Hendrick, 1994). In each of these areas the state was becoming more interventionist through legislation. Both the state and charitable welfare organizations were now making a number of assumptions mainly derived from the rise of 'psycho-medicine', about what constituted a proper childhood. There was a growing concern with children's rights and an assumption that it was the state alone that could enforce these rights (Cunningham, 1995). Protecting children and their rights was in harmony with the larger purposes of the state, which was of securing the reproduction of a society capable of competing in the harsh conditions of the twentieth century (Cunningham, 1995). These developments consolidated the idea that childhood is a period essentially different to adulthood and marked by vulnerability that required protection. Children in middle class Western society were viewed as approaching this new ideal for childhood, with other childhoods (for example in colonized countries) being seen as primitive and uncivilized.

The inter war period saw further significant refinements of the conceptualization of childhood through the influence of early developmental psychology and the birth of child psychiatry in the child guidance movement (Woolridge, 1995, Hendrick, 1994, 1997). A properly functioning family was deemed essential for mental health and the role of the mother in rearing emotionally balanced children was emphasized. Children were now being viewed through a more psychological lens with their inner life of emotions, fantasies, dreams, instincts and unconscious conflicts being explored. A more understanding, liberal and tolerant attitude towards children was encouraged by European professionals (Rose, 1985). By the 1930's child guidance clinics had become important propagandist institutions through radio talks, popular publications and lectures that promoted certain views of happy families and happy children which were dependent upon a new tolerance of and sympathy for the child (Rose, 1985)- a view that would finally catch the cultural imagination in the post-second world war West.

At this point in time medically dominated therapeutic institutions for children and adolescents were still a long way off as the dominant construction of childhood and its problems had yet to be viewed through a 'mental illness/psychiatric diagnosis' lens. However, increasing interest in the inner psychological life of children led to the creation of the first residential therapeutic communities in the UK and USA, set up on the ideals of self-government, greater permissiveness, psychological exploration and progressive education (e.g. the Caldecott community which was founded in 1911) (Bazeley, 1928). The growing impact of psychoanalysis led to new units being founded in 1930s Europe and North America for residential treatment of 'disturbed' children based on a combination of psychoanalytically based therapies and the development of a 'therapeutic milieu' (Whittaker, 1979).

Following the traumas of the Second World War and the evacuation process for children in Britain, prominence began to be given to the effects of early separation of young children from their mothers. This construction was reinforced by the development of attachment theory by the British psychoanalyst John Bowlby (1969, 1973). The evacuation was to reveal the extent of urban poverty and slum housing, the tenacity of ordinary working class families in sticking together and the existence of what was coming to be known as the 'problem family'. Evacuation, it was claimed, had shone a torchlight into the darkest corners of urban Britain and was revealing frightening implications for racial efficiency, emotional stability and post war democracy (MacNicol, 1986, Inglis, 1989 and Holman, 1995). Separation, it was now claimed, produced an affectionless character that was the root cause of anti-social behaviour (Bowlby 1969, 1973).

With the birth of the welfare state in the United Kingdom, citizens now had a right to free social and health services. This deliberate democratization of citizenship began with an eye on sustaining a healthy and growing population as well as a fear of the effects of the growth of communism throughout Europe and nationalism throughout the empire. New rights for children were enshrined in the Children Act of 1948 in Britain, which established local authority children's departments and emphasized a preference to boarding out children in foster families rather than residential homes, returning children in care to their natural parents and proceeding to adoption where appropriate. It also suggested that the publicly cared child should now be treated as an individual who had rights and possessions (Hendrick, 1994, 1997).

With the creation of the new National Health Service, the UK opened the first in-patient psychiatric department for children at the Maudsley hospital in 1947 (Cameron, 1949). Others soon followed. The new units emphasized broad investigation and assessment and a philosophy of 'total treatment' dealing with socio-psycho-biological aspects. Over the next few decades' big changes in the institutional response to childhood problems took place, reflecting changing cultural attitudes and conceptualizations with regards childhood and its problems.

Questions began to be asked about the quality and appropriateness of much institutional care offered to children. There resulted a steady decline in the number of children living in children's homes, a process affected by the anti-institutional movement warning about the adverse effect of institution-alization (Wolkind, 1974). Economic considerations came into play and a decline in therapeutic communities occurred during the 1980's as local authorities began to favour cheaper local alternatives. At the same time as non-medical therapeutic institutions were declining in number, medically funded in-patient adolescent units were expanding in number (Wardle, 1991). In the USA there was a burgeoning number of for profit, private residential treatment units with a doubling in the numbers of children in these units between 1969 and 1981, reflecting the increasing popularity (and financial reward offered) of using a psychiatric frame for childhood problems (Taube and Barrett, 1985).

In the UK psychiatric residential units at first tended to operate idiosyncratic approaches reflecting the beliefs of senior staff and local funding authorities, but by the mid-eighties a national set of standards was put in place whereby each region should have access to adequate numbers of beds on general purpose adolescent units that were capable of combining, short and long term and emergence functions (NHS Health Advisory Service, 1985). By now more eclectic models were being used to frame the approaches of the in-patient units with a trend of moving away from psychodynamic principles toward more behavioural ones with greater use of psychiatric diagnosis and medication (Parry-Jones, 1998).

The contemporary context:

The eighties and nineties saw the widespread establishment of right wing monetarist policies in Western economies and with it new economic controls on state health and welfare provisions at the same time as further individualizing ideals of growth, market expansion and wealth creation. This had a profound effect on the managed healthcare system in the USA. With the managed healthcare system being the bread and butter of the majority of psychiatrists and paediatrician's work, when the more labour intensive psychotherapies lost favour with healthcare insurers, doctors soon realized they could make more money by going down the psychopharmacology route than the psychotherapy one- Much more. Doctors can earn three times more by 15 minute medication review follow ups than a 45 minute visit with the child's family. Managed healthcare has meant an economic system has come to be built around DSM IV diagnoses, with diagnoses offering an easy way to organize the economic system of psychiatric healthcare. In order to obtain a legitimate ticket to a service, you need a DSM IV diagnosis. Thus DSM IV has become a more than a mental health diagnostic manual; it is a legal, financial and ideological document, driving thinking about all sorts of emotions and behaviours, including those of our children toward ever more medicalized notions.

The greater medicalization of American child and adolescent psychiatry together with its cultural power has resulted in child psychiatry in the UK itself changing enormously in the last 10 years. Thus the UK's professional discourse has similarly become convinced that there are more personal and professional rewards to be gained by it adopting a more medicalized American style approach (e.g. Goodman, 1997). This has helped construct the field of neuro-developmental psychiatry, which the public, trusting such high status opinions, has come to view as real.

Paralleling these developments within child and adolescent psychiatry has been, not surprisingly, similar developments within residential child and adolescent psychiatry settings. In the USA this has resulted in the widespread adoption of the 'brief hospitalization' model of intervention, whereby patients are admitted for relatively short periods- typically around a month (after which health insurance often runs out) for diagnostic assessment and psychopharmacological interventions. Whilst UK units still offer varied therapeutic interventions in most adolescent in-patient psychiatric residential units, the hierarchical structure means that diagnosis and medical (usually pharmacological) interventions assume the greatest organising influence on the philosophical approach of current UK units.

In conclusion then the nature of residential adolescent in-patient units can be understood as being a product of the social/political/economic/cultural conditions within which they exist. Just as each development can be situated within in its own historical context so the current situation doesn't represent some sort of end-point and is likely to change as a result of social dynamics such as changing economic, political and medical opinion.

Changing the culture at Ash Villa:

Following our (the two authors, ST and EM) arrival at Ash Villa in 2002 we began to the slow, challenging and often stressful task of trying to move the guiding philosophy at Ash Villa away from the medical model as an organizing principle and toward new ways of context-rich thinking that reflected recent developments in theory and practice (such as those detailed in other chapters in this book). Ash Villa is a 12-bedded regional general adolescent mental health in-patient unit taking young people between the ages of 10 and 18 for all types of mental health difficulties that require in-patient treatment. We found that there were two main issues that required some thought and understanding.

The problems:

The first issue confronting us was that the unit had functioned within a medical model framework and hierarchy for many years and the staff understood their role as being within this. One of the authors (EM) own experience of traditional nurse training (pre Project 2000 nurse training syllabus) and clinical practice had, in the main, fallen within the realms of the medical model. Her experience was that this way of working formed the guiding principles for practise within all fields of mental health with which she had thus far worked or came into contact with. The hospital environment was no exception and in her training she had been taught to recognise signs and symptoms of mental illness and how to manage these through supporting medical interventions. The other author's (ST) previous experience of working on or coming into contact with adolescent psychiatric in-patient units in the UK was also that these are now dominated by medical model thinking with most patients receiving some form of psychotropic medication. In addition, prior to our arrival in early 2002, the unit had undergone a long period of instability. There had been several changes in Consultant Psychiatrist over the previous few years and the unit had suffered other staffing difficulties. Nursing staff levels were low and there was a feeling of exhaustion amongst the existing staff, with their energy going into surviving and keeping the unit open to admissions. Many of the staff were feeling de-skilled and undervalued through not being able to develop consistent therapeutic work with the young people and their families, their role often being little more than babysitters for the doctors.

Secondly, within Ash Villa (and the mental health service more generally), the nursing process offered an individualised approach to care that followed a rigid linear system (derived from medical model thinking) of assessment, plan, implementation and evaluation. The focus of the care plan was problem centred leaving very little scope within the planning process for looking at, and building upon, existing strengths of the young person and their family. Therefore, the unit ethos revolved around a focus on getting rid of problems with little emphasis on building on the positives.

Although we perceived the above two issues as our priority issues to tackle, there were, other 'cultural' problems that confronted us. Many families arrived with an understanding that they were unable to cope and were often reluctant to engage in therapeutic family work. Family work was taking place on the unit, however it was infrequent, on an ad hoc basis by staff with an interest in family work, did not feature within the regular structure of the unit, had a marginal status, and rarely informed a process dominated by a narrow medical perspective. This lack of a more systemic perspective was reinforcing the idea that 'professionals' or 'experts' can cope more effectively than the family, who were then inadvertently forced (or relieved) to take a 'back seat'. The marginal status of the broader perspective, further strengthened the idea that the difficulties the young person admitted to Ash Villa was presenting with, were best understood as a product of the internal goings on in that child's brain (a potentially disabling belief that could persist for many years after discharge) as well as causing missed possibilities for solutions that can be found within the much wider context of the family and community.

Another issue relates to the effects of the system pre-admission and post-discharge. When young people are admitted to Ash Villa, the system and process has often compounded the 'ill child' scenario. By the time the young person has been admitted they have already been seen by a child and adolescent psychiatrist within a medical hierarchy organized community child and adolescent mental health service (CAMHS), there is often more than one agency involved (for example social services and education as well as CAMHS), they have at least one diagnostic label (many cases have several diagnoses), and are taking at least one type of psychotropic medication (many cases more than one). By being referred to a 'psychiatric unit' such as Ash Villa, the young person and their family have often understandably already internalized a feeling that many people think they (the referred young person) must be terribly ill. Once young people are discharged, their care is usually returned to the same, usually medically orientated CAMHS that first referred them.

Changing the institutional culture:

Our arrival at Ash Villa in early 2002 coincided with several changes in nursing staff and other new appointments (such as a part-time psychotherapist and part-time staff grade doctor). Our task was helped greatly by this new injection of enthusiasm for change, with staff who were generally sympathetic to our thinking. Like many institutions in the UK National Health Service (NHS), we were aware that there was a certain amount of 'change fatigue' following changes within the structure of the local health authority and the employing NHS trust, as well as the unit having to survive the recent instability, and so initially we worked within the existing structures at Ash Villa with change being introduced slowly and in relation to our management of individual cases in the first instance.

Some conflicts were inevitable. Although non-medical staff are usually more open to alternative, more psychotherapeutic, models of working, weaning young people off medication caused some staff great anxiety, having been used to using medication to manage challenging behaviour. Although most were, in principle, in favour of reducing our reliance on medication, this also meant nursing staff having to get used to managing a higher level of challenging behaviour, a process that was stressful, uncomfortable and often resulted in conflicts between some staff and those of us in the more senior roles who were trying to change the unit's cultural approach to such difficulties.

Another source of early conflicts was with other agencies involved, particularly social services. At the time of our arrival at Ash Villa, the unit was full and local consultants had to refer some of their patients to out of county in-patient units, due to this. There was an attitude around that once a young person was admitted to Ash Villa, their problems were 'mental health' and nothing to do with social services. A number of the young people on the unit at that time had been there for a considerable period of time and the issues keeping them at Ash Villa were more social than health (such as parental neglect). As with many other parts of the country, the local social services were struggling financially and were reluctant to get involved in helping young people at Ash Villa who may need to go into the care system, as they were deemed to be in a 'place of safety' whilst at Ash Villa. Sadly, this meant having to force the system to respond in some cases by notifying social services that a discharge date had been arranged, as the young person concerned was no longer needing health input and that we believed that they would be at risk of 'child abuse' should they return home. This caused conflicts that resulted in top-level management of both health and social services having to become involved resulting in some changes in the ways our services work together and the successful discharge of young people who had been inappropriately placed at Ash Villa. This process together with changes in our admissions protocol has meant that we have not had a problem with bed availability since those early months.

We also needed to find a way to work co-operatively with local CAMHS. We decided that our first priority was to develop our own strong and coherent identity and develop our relationships with local services from this platform. When we first arrived, local CAMHS consultants were helping manage their own patients who had been admitted to Ash Villa, in order to help manage the shortage of consistent consultant cover for the unit. This arrangement continued for a good month after our arrival, with one of the authors (ST) gradually taking over consultant responsibility. After this 'settling in' period we deliberately changed the day and structure of the weekly case discussion meeting and took complete ownership of the cases at Ash Villa. From there we discussed with the local CAMHS consultants what they would like from us, and how we could maintain good communication/contact with them whilst their patients were at Ash Villa. This led in time to several developments such as 24hour, 7day a week access to Ash Villa for urgent admissions from the community (keeping an emergency bed available at all times, as far as possible), and an admissions process that involved an early review meeting with the referring CAMHS, other relevant agencies, the young person and their family/carers, followed by regular 6 weekly review meetings with all the above. Local CAMHS are now aware of our therapeutic orientation and although this has led to some disagreements we appear to have developed a healthy respect for each others ways of working, which has enabled some of the local consultants to use our orientation to help out with cases where the medical approach is stuck (for example we have had several referrals for cases with diagnoses such as ADHD were our work has been to wean the young person off medication that was not helping and to re-conceptualise their difficulties in non-medical terms).

Making such changes also challenges the medical hierarchy of the employing trust. Although senior management within our trust have been sympathetic to and supportive of our efforts to develop a more positive and psychotherapeutic climate at Ash Villa, institionalised systems sometimes result in difficult to resolve conflicts. For example, the trust database requires us to input a diagnostic code for each young person admitted. This clashed with our desire to move away from single word diagnoses as an organizing principle for our approach. Initially we simply refused to input a code. When pressured to do so we started inputting the 'no diagnosis' code. This led to a heated discussion with those managing the database about how a psychiatric unit could be admitting patients with no diagnosis. One of the author's (ST) reply to this was that it was because at Ash Villa we inevitably admit those at the more complex end of the spectrum of clinical difficulties for whom 'one word formulations' is not useful. This issue remains unresolved.

Another area of difficulty relates to the large and seemingly never ending documents on trust policies and procedures which are often motivated by self-protection on the part of the trust and can constrain creative therapeutic work. For example, the trust policy on absconding necessitated staff to follow a young person, search for them and eventually call the police. Whilst this was appropriate for some young people, for others it proved reinforcing and sometimes we would overhear a young person bragging to their peers about the thrill of the chase and outwitting the staff. Furthermore, institutional responses are often rather concrete and can alienate staff from thinking about the meaning of the behaviour and finding more creative approaches. Moving thinking beyond a 'policies and procedures' mentality has helped develop more creative ideas. One young lad on the unit used to repeatedly abscond, and we worked out that this was in part due to his wanting to be on his own when feelings got unbearable. As a way forward, we encouraged him to build a 'den' within the grounds of Ash Villa where he could retreat to when he needed to be alone.

Having begun the process of change through a gradual change in the management of individual cases, it was time to look at our overall structure and ethos. A series of development days was arranged to include all disciplines on the unit. This was the first opportunity for the nursing, medical, therapy, teaching, administration and housekeeping staff to meet together for a full day to share their visions, discuss the successes (as well as the problems) of the unit and agree a way forward. On these development days, the young people on the unit would spend an extra day at home (where possible) to enable all staff to attend.

As part of our development work we discussed the unit philosophy that will guide our clinical approach, eventually developing a kind of mission statement to reflect our attitude: '*At Ash Villa we believe in supporting the well being of young people in their families – Building on courage, knowledge and strengths.*' Our orientation toward a more 'health building' rather than 'problem eliminating' framework has had several knock on effects. For example, the school at Ash Villa has been enthused to become a more active participant in the overall therapeutic programme. They have become actively involved in the national 'healthy schools initiative' which has resulted in more active forms of teaching to engage the young people, including weekly educational outings (recent examples include learning horse riding and sailing), the re-design of the school garden including natural sculptures made by the young people, and the establishment of a small organic vegetable garden. The school also obtained funding to build the now completed 'trim trail' in the Ash Villa grounds. The teachers are now regular contributors to all clinical meetings and case reviews working closely with the young people's main school to enable successful re-integrations back to them.

The development days also helped us build up a more coherent therapeutic timetable involving all the clinical staff. Our clinical therapeutic focus (as our unit philosophy statement suggests) understands the young person within their wider context. It is now a unit expectation that family therapy/work will take place on a regular basis with the families/carers of every young person admitted to Ash Villa. As well as formal family therapy, we try other creative ways of involving the family, for example inviting parents of young people with eating problems to join us at mealtimes and using telephone advice to deal with crises when a young person is on leave. The systemic focus goes beyond the family and we expect professionals from other involved agencies to attend regular meetings. In addition individual work occurs in the form of art therapy, psychotherapy and key-worker input, as well as group approaches (recent examples include a relaxation group, a self-esteem group, a shiatsu group and a music group).

The unit needed a great deal of support in managing the difficulties arising from the intensive cases. At one particularly difficult time, the average age group of the young people resident on the unit was 15 to 17 years old with most of these young people presenting with challenging and high-risk behaviours, such as deliberate self-harm. Not surprisingly, the conflict from within the young people was creating conflict within the staff group. The staff experienced a sense of despair and a feeling of 'not coping' that echoed a process that young people and their families were struggling with.

Behaviours such as deliberate self-harm can be extremely stressful for staff teams and our systems often try to by-pass the human emotions that are stirred up, by 'technicalising' our responses through use of impersonal constructs such 'risk'. Clinical Governance within health services includes everyone having to develop policies and procedures for 'risk management'. In more ordinary human terms however, there is a fine line between managing risk in a safe and effective way and becoming an over-anxious health professional protecting ones own back by trying to over-zealously prevent risk. When a young person was deliberately self-harming, it was common practice at Ash Villa, to search rooms for sharp objects to try and prevent this from happening again. The 'what if' . . . question would be raised and this would lead the staff trying to take control of the situation and removing any harmful objects. Yet we know that in the majority of cases, people use self-harm as a coping strategy. Stopping this may then leave the person without any meaningful strategy to them, which, paradoxically, may well increase the risk for that person.

We decided some new thinking might be helpful. The management of deliberate self-harm was discussed with the team, the young person and the family, so that agreement was reached on how to manage any incidences. Following this we began to work with each young person and their family/ carer, to explore alternative, safer coping strategies. An important component to this was family work to try and foster new ways of understanding these behaviours and how to manage them. The result of going through this process has, in general, been that staff are now less anxious and more tolerant of self-harm behaviours. Young people are encouraged to inform staff of their desire to self-harm before they do so, however, if they do, we try not to make too much of a 'fuss' about it and encourage the young person to clean and dress any wounds themselves. By using such an approach, of not making a therapeutic issue of the self-harm, our experience has been that many of our client's self-harming behaviour has diminished and then stopped of its own accord.

Issues such as self-harm, that cause allot of anxiety within the staff group, forced us to think about helping staff manage the difficult feelings that were now being stirred up as we sought to develop an ethos around engagement with and acceptance of, human uncertainty. We therefore decided to start having a weekly staff meeting where staff are encouraged to discuss the difficulties they are required to manage, and the feelings these evoke. Although this is a well-recognized component of many therapeutic communities, it was new to a staff group who had been working within the medical model framework previously used on the unit. Some of these meetings were extremely difficult and there were some uncomfortable and stressful battles. However, the meetings enabled the staff to explore and challenge their own and others assumptions, share ideas and reach agreements on how to manage difficulties and it soon became a forum where our therapeutic framework could begin to be re-formulated.

For example, there were instances when some of our clients were perceived to reject any attempts to engage therapeutically. For some of them, this was probably part of an attempt to 'test' the staff's ability to stick with them, before they felt that it was worth the emotional investment. This created strong feelings within the staff team. Staff would experience frustration and would question whether the young person should remain on the unit if they were unwilling to engage. Through discussions, heated 'battles' and frank exchanges in the staff meetings, new ways of understanding this 'lack of engagement' was developed and more therapeutic 'patience' with the pace of change as well as more realistic goals for an admission began to be formulated. The team increased their understanding in the skill of being able to 'contain' and 'hold' clients and their families for long enough periods of time to enable a young person to 'move on'. The staff had now started to explore and develop new ideas about their own practice within the new ethos of the unit. They began to see, recognize and value the relationships they already had with the young people, where previously they may have been unaware of this value, as it was not specific structured work. Regular feedback for all staff soon became crucial so that the relationships between the young people and staff (whether positive or negative) was recognized and acknowledged by them as an important aspect of their work to be thought about, reflected upon and developed.

Case example:

Jayne was 15 years old when she was admitted urgently to the unit. Prior to her admission, Jayne was being treated for 'depression' and the referring consultant felt that Jayne was now developing a 'paranoid psychoses'. Jayne had a recent history of aggressive behaviour, deliberate self-harm, non-school attendance and fear of leaving the family home; believing people were 'looking at her' and 'talking about her'. Jayne had been given various antidepressant and antipsychotic medications over the preceding weeks and months however, despite this she continued to deteriorate.

Jayne and her family came to the unit with the script that Jayne was ill and that they, as a family, were unable to cope with her illness, which they felt needed professionals to properly 'treat' it. Following her admission to the unit, Jayne would attempt to scratch her arms and bang her head against the wall. This was distressing for the family who would hold Jayne's arms to stop her doing this. Jayne confined herself to her room on the unit, insisting that she couldn't cope with being outside a very small-circumscribed area on the unit. On admission Jayne was taking an antidepressant and an antipsychotic. These were both weaned off and discontinued within the first few weeks of admission (as has been the case with nearly all those admitted on psychotropic medication, since our arrival at Ash Villa).

Jayne was initially nursed under close observations to prevent her from harming herself. However, this exacerbated Jayne's dependency on others, and so we began to encourage the staff to start encouraging and sometimes insisting that Jayne takes some responsibility for her behaviour (for example by refusing to escort her to the nearby bathroom). We discussed Jayne's self-harming behaviour and all agreed that the nursing staff would now stop intervening when Jayne went to bang her head or scratch her arms. Staff were extremely anxious about this fearing the level of damage that Jayne might inflict upon herself. They supported each other in assessing each situation as it arose and within days, Jayne stopped banging her head against the wall. The scratching and cutting reduced from daily to happening at times of stress (often around the 6 weekly case review meeting, were the Jayne's anxiety was about whether she may be discharged).

Jayne, along with the staff, became more able to identify the times when she was more at risk of self-harming and she began to share with us how she was feeling, rather than always acting this out. Family work/therapy took place mainly at the family's home where the parents' model of understanding Jayne's behaviour was discussed and new ways of managing Jayne's difficulties at home were suggested. Jayne's parents became more confident in their parenting ability and also took began taking steps to withdraw from constantly trying to stop her harming herself. Jayne's parents were also encouraged to start examining their own lives, which had come revolve around 'caring' for their 'ill' daughter in a mutually reinforcing negative cycle. As a result Jayne's father became more able to allow Jayne's mother to manage Jayne without him, and Jayne's mother started looking for and then attending adult education classes for herself.

As time went on and Jayne's behaviour began to settle she started spending more time at home. However, from time to time Jayne still became distressed and distressing and during one of these particularly difficult times on the unit, Jayne's parents were contacted and asked to take her home and manage her there for a few days. This proved to be an important turning point. Up until this moment, much of the few months work on the unit had been broadly that of containment, with us taking the lead to change our responses in order to move Jayne out of what we considered to be excessive dependency. We maintained daily telephone contact on this occasion and the family managed the situation extremely well without having to bring Jayne back earlier than agreed (as had been happening previously). The family's ideas about their coping abilities had changed and for the first time, they had demonstrated genuine confidence in their ability to manage and cope with a difficult rather than ill teenager. On her return Jayne started to take some control and responsibility for managing her distress. No longer were we having to do the 'weaning' off of her dependency, she was now motivated to do this herself. She began taking a lead role in some of the groups on the unit and was for the first time requesting more time at home. The staff and Jayne's family encouraged her interests in music and fashion and she began to develop a much clearer, age appropriate self-identity. Jayne was successfully discharged some weeks later and follow-up outreach visits showed that Jayne and her family were now flourishing.

Conclusion

In this chapter we have reviewed the history of the 'institutional' child to demonstrate that our institutional response to childhood deviance reflects the historical and cultural context of the time. Our current responses, to childhood deviance must also be considered as being historically and culturally embedded and likely to change as our ideas about the nature and cause of problematic behaviours change.

We then explored the process of change that has taken place at an adolescent in-patient unit in which we hold senior positions. The example from this unit is to demonstrate that alternatives to the current dominant construction used in most British adolescent mental health in-patient units (the medical model), is possible despite all the systemic constraints against this. Furthermore, the importance of challenging the hegemony of medicalization is not only to demonstrate that positive outcomes can and do occur without it (there is little evidence to suggest that medicalized units produce any long term benefit), but also for the subtler cultural reason of showing that even those psychiatry would consider the most 'ill' can be liberated in a helpful way from such a hope crushing self-definitions. This challenges some the central cherished assumptions of Western child and adolescent psychiatry.

Acknowledgements

A big thank you to all the staff at Ash Villa and all the clients who have taught us so much and a special thank you to those clients who consented to their stories being used.

References

Baistow, K. (1995) From sickly survival to realisation of potential: Child health as a social project. *Children in Society* 9, 20-35.

Bowlby, J. (1969) *Attachment and Loss, Volume 1, Attachment.* London: Hogarth Press.

Bowlby, J. (1973) *Attachment and Loss, Volume 2, Separation.* London: Hogarth Press.

Carpenter, M. (1853) *Juvenile Delinquents: Their Condition and Treatment.* London: Cash.

Cunningham, H. (1991) *The Children of the Poor: Representations of Childhood Since the Seventeenth Century.* Oxford: Basil Blackwell.

Cunningham, H. (1995) *Children and Childhood in Western Society Since 1500.* London: Longman.

Davidoff, L. and Hall, C. (1987) *Family Fortunes: Men and Women of the English Middle Class 1788-1850.* London: Hutchinson.

Foucault M. (1971) *Madness and Civilization: a History of Insanity in the Age of Reason.* London: Tavistock.

Goodman, R. (1997) An over extended remit. *British Medical Journal* 314, 813-814.

Hendrick, H. (1992) Changing attitudes to children 1800-1914. *Genealogists Magazine* 24, 41-9.

Hendrick, H. (1994) *Child Welfare England 1870-1989.* London: Routledge.

Hendrick, H. (1997) 'Constructions and reconstructions of British childhood: An interpretive survey, 1800 to the present' in A. James and A. Prout (eds.) *Constructing and Reconstructing Childhood: Contemporary Issues in the Sociological Study of Childhood.* London: Falmer Press.

Holman, B. (1995) *The Evacuation.* London: The Lion Press.

Humphries, S. (1981) *Hooligans or Rebels? An Oral History of Working Class Childhood and Youth, 1889-1939.* Oxford: Blackwell.

Inglis, R. (1989) *The Children's War: Evacuation 1939-45.* London: Fontana.

La Fontaine, J.S. (1979) *Sex and Age as Principles of Social Differentiation.* London: Academic Press.

MacNicol, J. (1986) 'The effect of the evacuation of school children on official attitudes to state intervention' in H.L. Smith (ed.) *War And Social Change: British Society In The Second World War.* Manchester: Manchester University Press.

Manton, J. (1976) *Mary Carpenter And The Children Of The Street.* London: Heinemann.

May, M. (1973) Innocence and experience in the evolution of the concept of juvenile delinquency in the mid-nineteenth century. *Victorian Studies* 17, 7-29.

Pearson, G. (1983) *Hooligan: A History of Respectable Fears.* London: MacMillan.

Pincbeck, I. And Hewitt, M. (1973) *Children in English Society.* London: Routledge and Kegan Paul.

Porter R. (1987) *A Social History of Madness: Stories of the Insane.* London: Weidenfeld and Nicolson.

Prout, A. and James, A. (1997) 'A new Paradigm for the sociology of childhood? Provenance, promise and problems' in A. James and A. Prout (eds.) *Constructing And Re-Constructing Childhood: Contemporary Issues In The Sociological Study Of Childhood.* London: Falmer Press.

Rose, N. (1985) *The Psychological Complex: Psychology, Politics and Society in England 1869-1939.* London: RKP.

Rothman, D. (1984) *Evangelicals and Culture.* London: Croom Helm.

Selleck, R.J.W. (1985) Mary Carpenter: A confident and contradictory reformer. *History of Education* March, 101-15.

Sutherland, G. (1984) *Ability, Merit And Measurement Mental Testing And English Education.* Oxford: Clarendon Press.

Taube C. and Barret, S.A. (1985) *Mental Health in the United States, 1985.* Rockville: National Institute of Mental Health.

Wooldridge, A. (1995) *Measuring the Mind.* Cambridge: Cambridge University Press.

Zelizer, V.A. (1985) *Pricing The Priceless Child: The Changing Social Value Of Children.* New York: Basic Books Inc.

8
Systemic Approaches – critique and scope

Eia Asen

Systemic practice – past and present

The term 'systemic' is now much in use, covering a whole range of different activities and models. Adopting systemic perspectives means viewing the child and his or her mental issues in a variety of contexts. These include not only the immediate and the wider family, but also the social and cultural setting of which the child and family are part. A systemic perspective also includes examining the relationship between the child, the family and the professional 'team' that constructs and/or diagnoses 'mental health issues' or psychiatric illness or disorder. Professional networks are 'problem-generated systems' and they develop with overt, as well as covert agenda, reflecting the wider political contexts and their ever-changing priorities.

The field of family therapy hi-jacked the term 'systemic' many years ago when the family was described, somewhat mechanistically, as a 'system' with different 'parts' (the family members). The notion of the family as a system is both useful and problematic. Problematic as it, at best, can only serve as a metaphor and should not be mistaken for something 'real'. Useful, as the use of the concept can have clinical implications describing families – and related systems – as possessing homeostatic tendencies and a variety of 'properties', such as hierarchies, boundaries, sub-groups, as well as overt and covert communication exchanges between specific members, coalitions, and so on. For clinicians it can be useful to see family members as behaving according to a set of explicit and implicit rules (however speculative), developed over time and often over generations, which govern their relationships and communications (Watzlawick et al 1967). If such rules can be uncovered or discovered, and if they are believed to contribute to the presenting problems, then this has pragmatic implications for change: the rules can be questioned and challenged and new interaction can emerge. Furthermore, systems theory claims that changing just one part of the system (the patient's symptoms, for example) results in changes elsewhere (communications). This also has pragmatic implications for change and the anthropologist G. Bateson and his team (Bateson et al 1956) first applied systems ideas to patients 'with' schizophrenia. They 'found' the patient's distorted thought processes were the result of the family's complex and contradictory transaction and communication patterns. Born was the 'identified patient' – identified and perhaps even victimized by the 'system', which could be the family or the larger oppressive political system. It did not take long before clinicians 'observed' that if the 'identified patient' improved, the rest of the family could become destabilised, adding seemingly further 'proof' that some families could be 'toxic' or 'schizophrenogenic' (Laing & Esterson 1971).

These clinicians and their followers postulated that the family needed the patient to remain unwell, therefore blocking, if not fighting against, the clinical improvement of the patient. Within that frame it seemed logical that if individual pathology developed within the family, then its very breeding ground needed to be treated: the family. The early family therapy pioneers had a tendency to blame the family for the illness or problems of their offspring. Not surprisingly, family therapy was therefore at the outset not very popular – and particularly not with families. It also was not particularly 'systemic' as the thinking was very much embedded in the medical model: instead of genes 'causing' schizophrenia, it became the family that was seen as the cause of it all.

In fact, the very term 'family therapy' was – and remains – rather controversial and may be misleading. Is it not the case that, if asked, most families would decline the offer of being 'therap-ed'?! The term 'therapy' implies the presence of illness or dysfunction, located in a person or the family, rather than beyond those boundaries. It is a politically sanctioned concept in that it puts blame for 'dysfunction' at the door of the individual or family rather than linking it to prevailing social realities and inequalities. And, what's more, does one need to be a family to receive this treatment? Family forms have changed since the systemic approach was born more than half a century ago. No longer is the two-parent, heterosexual couple with their 'own' children the norm. In many countries we now have many families with single parents, or children living in gay or lesbian relationships or communes, we have reconstituted families, as wells as children and teenagers living in other forms of committed relationships and friendships. Family therapists have had to continuously re-examine their assumptions, presumptions and practices and to change in line with evolving new societal practices and realities. Furthermore, in the wake of globalization and economic migration, as well as a result of wars that have led to the displacement of millions of families, most clinicians have become increasingly confronted with families from other cultures, presenting with very different, culture-specific and often religion-based, belief systems. Family therapists have had to acknowledge that their theories are essentially Eurocentric and that new models of practice needed to be evolved, learning from differences, rather than making different cultural practices fit into their Westernised models and interventions.

As a result systemic practice has changed considerably over the past half century. Its focus has also shifted, away from an early interest in families containing adult schizophrenic members, to working with families containing problematic children and adolescents – and problematic parents (Minuchin et al 1964, Haley 1979). Systemic practice has also developed in very different contexts, some private and some public, and changing political realities have led to specific systemic approaches. The early pioneers (e.g. Ackerman 1966) were preoccupied with unconscious processes and the structural therapists (Minuchin 1974, Minuchin & Fishman 1981) largely replaced psychoanalytical ideas with a rather concrete but also pragmatic model. Their preoccupation with allegedly 'dysfunctional' hierarchies between the generations, or 'inadequate' boundaries between parents and their children, reflected normative ideas and prejudices which prevailed then, with some of the resulting interventions coming close to a mild form of social engineering.

Another school of thought, the strategic family therapists (Haley 1963, Watzlawick et al 1974) aimed to deliver interventions, or 'strategies', to fit the presenting problems. One of the underlying assumptions of the approach was that the illness – or problem – was being maintained by the apparent 'solution', namely the very behaviour(s) that sought to reduce the problem. The strategic therapists produced some imaginative interventions, with at times seemingly outrageous re-frames, some of which resembled the emerging 'trickery' employed so successfully by American salesmen, and nowadays barely compatible with the authenticity and transparency desired by most clinicians working with children and families. Yet, the approach was also a welcome shift, away from the medical model, to putting 'illness' into different meaning frames.

The early Milan systemic approach (Selvini Palazzoli et al 1978) used elements but, being European in essence and initially psychoanalytically influenced, attempted to go 'deeper'. It focused on family patterns that were thought to have evolved over generations and that seemed to organise family life in the present. Families with entrenched intra-familial interaction styles were believed to have a tendency to disqualify therapists and the Milan team specialised in the treatment of these 'intractable' families, designing interventions, which took into account the anticipated attempts of the family to disqualify the therapeutic ventures. The resulting 'counter-paradoxes' prescribed by the team can be thought of as strategic manoeuvres, in that by recommending 'no change' the therapist hoped that the family would resist this command and do the opposite, namely change – if only to defeat the therapist!

Paradoxical prescriptions were fashionable in the 1980s but are rarely used nowadays, as they do not fit with the emerging climate of openness and transparency and of involving service users centrally in their recovery. Furthermore, the prescription of a ritual to the family, 'ex cathedra' as it were, in the expectation that they will defy it, can be seen as mocking and patronizing. However, what has survived from the early Milan approach is a particular style of interviewing which in itself is an intervention: circular and reflexive questioning (Selvini Palazzoli et al 1980). In addition, the Milan team's commitment to 'positive connotation' has produced a non-blaming approach which is still embraced by many systemic practitioners: the actions of all family members are primarily seen as the best everyone could do under the circumstances – even if the outcome of family members' actions were seemingly negative, the intentions are viewed as positive. Clearly such a relativistic approach also has its limitations and can meet with considerable resistance, particular amongst professional subscribing to bio-medical frameworks. Furthermore, the – then – insistence on the position of 'neutrality' of the therapist often seemed a rather unethical stance to adopt, particularly for those CAMHS workers involved in child protection work. The stance of 'neutrality' has subsequently been replaced by 'curiosity' (Cecchin 1987) that seems more practicable and acceptable.

Psycho-educational approaches (Leff et al 1982, Anderson 1983, Kuipers et al 1992) have found their particular application in the field of adult psychiatry and especially in the work with psychotic patients and their families. This model tends to be used when working with the carers of mentally ill family members, teaching them about the 'illness' and its causes and the 'best' way of responding to and managing the ill person. One aspect of this approach is to reduce the levels of the carers' Expressed Emotion (Vaughn & Leff 1976) and particularly the amount of critical comments, hostility and over-involvement they show towards the 'identified' patient. This approach is less relevant to clinicians working with children and teenagers. However, the concept of Expressed Emotion (EE), so strongly associated with psycho-educational approaches, has now almost become a fetish, worshipped by the scientific community and thus requires brief further discussion.

Is EE real or is 'it' merely a social construction? And, if it really is real, should we then not make it our primary business to reduce EE in parents? Should we not be teaching parents how to show 'warmth' to their children and how to avoid being over-critical of, hostile to and over-involved with one's offspring? If put like this it is difficult to classify psycho-educational approaches as being systemic, since they tend to specialize in linear and somewhat hydraulic interventions, rather than permitting clinicians to bathe in our much-loved circular epistemologies. Systemic practitioners can at times be quite dismissive of psycho-educational models, but in practice many clinicians who work in CAMHS settings may deliberately or inadvertently borrow some of these techniques, particularly when families insist that one of their members has a real 'illness' (psychological or physical). Sticking with such a frame can help to engage families – and the parents in particular – as they do not find their own 'diagnosis' disconfirmed.

The most recent phase in the development of systemic therapy has been influenced by the social constructionist approach (Gergen 1994, Flaskas 2002). It is in marked contrast to biomedical models, in that it deconstructs the notion that there is an objective reality 'out there'. Instead, social constructionists believe that the 'reality' therapists observe is 'invented', with perceptions being shaped by the therapists' own cultures, their implicit assumptions and beliefs and the language they use to describe things. The notion of the 'problem-determined' system (Anderson et al 1986) refers to how interactions between clinicians and clients or families are programmed by the built-in assumptions inherent in the traditional clinical discourses employed to discuss experiences and relationships. As long as therapeutic encounters focus on clients' experiences as evidence of illness or pathology, they remain trapped in pathology frames. By contrast, if one subscribes to the view that each culture has its own and specific dominant narratives and discourses (Foucault 1975), then one is led to question the medically dominated narratives Western cultures have invented to explain, simplify and categorise the complex problems of living which many families experience. If the narratives in which children have their experience 'storied' by others do not fit their own 'reality', then significant aspects of their lived experience will contradict the dominant narrative (White & Epston 1990) and be experienced as problematic. Clinicians' narratives – and the implied assumptions – may be experienced as being 'alien' or powerful, so much so that they take over the consultation.

This can amount to a distancing expert stance, very different from being curious and led by the child's narrative and aiming to develop a shared new narrative. This way of thinking has led to an examination of how language shapes problem perceptions and definitions (Goolishian & Anderson 1987). The very term 'problem' can be problematic, as can be the term 'solution', possibly promising a 'quick fix' when there are no quick solutions in sight. Systemic narrative therapy (White & Epston 1990) aims to enable clients and families to generate and evolve new stories, as well as finding ways of interpreting past and present events to make sense of their experiences. In this model the therapeutic process is seen as a mutually validating conversation, between patient and clinician, from which change can occur. They 'co-evolve' or 'co-construct' new ways of describing their own issues and family or couple dynamics, so that these no longer need to be viewed or experienced as problematic. Clinicians practicing in this way tend to describe themselves as being even-handed and realistic about the possibility of change, with no wish to impose their own ideas, being alert to openings as well as remaining curious about their own position in the observed system, taking non-judgmental and multi-positional stances (Jones 1993). Quite a task!!

Central to this approach is the process of reflection, which is seen – as it is in other approaches – as necessary to promote change. The 'reflecting team' (Andersen 1987) is one of the major innovations in recent years. No longer are there discussions between clinician and team members behind the one-way screen that exclude clients, but these conversations take place openly in front of the family. The implied sharing of the clinicians' thinking with clients involves the latter in a process of reflection rather than imposing interventions on them.

Brief 'solution focused' therapy (De Shazer 1985), interestingly and perhaps significantly emerged during the Reagan and Thatcher years, reflecting those politicians' obsession with being 'deaf' to problems and with almost compulsively looking for alleged solutions. This approach was a welcome departure from pathology dominated models as solution focused therapists deliberately ignore 'problem saturated' ways of talking and focus instead on the patterns of previous attempted solutions. The approach is based on the observation that symptoms and problems have a tendency to fluctuate. Concentrating on those times when a symptom, such as an anxiety state, is less or not present, allows the therapist to design therapeutic strategies around the exceptions, as they form the basis of the solution. The theory has it that by encouraging families to amplify the 'solution' patterns of their lives, the problem patterns can be driven into the background.

This account of past and current systemic practice and its origins is by necessity brief. Different schools and approaches have evolved slowly and steadily over the years, reflecting changing societal, cultural and political landscapes. Thankfully most systemic practitioners have left behind their 'teenage' battles as to which approach is 'best'. As systemic practice nears a more mature age, multi-modal collaboration and attempted integration of different systemic approaches and techniques are common. Practitioners have discovered that there are more similarities than differences between the various approaches. Moreover, by working in multi-cultural settings, clinicians are learning that families from different ethnic and religious backgrounds require different interventions. Most systemic therapists working in public services adapt their approach to the work contexts and presenting problems. It is accepted that different phases of therapy require different techniques, styles and positions of the therapist and different working contexts clearly require different responses to the patients and the problems they and their families present. It has been a positive development that most CAMHS settings now employ systemic therapists and that managers can see the value of such professionals as a useful addition to multi-disciplinary teams.

Systemic practitioners, as other mental health professionals, are under considerable pressure to prove that their approaches work. The emerging powerful force of 'evidence based medicine' (Sackett et al 1996) can be experienced as an unwelcome visitor and pressure, with its emphasis on outcomes being scientifically evaluated and an insistence that appropriate treatments need to be matched to specific conditions. This is a challenge to all those therapists who remain 'married' to just one specific brand of therapy, no matter what the patient's condition.

However, this condition-based evaluation, with its emphasis on reducing the complexity of human experience and suffering to a diagnosable label and to prescribing 'fitting' remedies, does have serious limitations. It tempts the main-stream clinicians who have much (political) interest to prove that 'their' method is best, with the less tested – though possibly no less effective – approaches increasingly becoming displaced from the 'shopping window' of an allegedly 'modern' and possibly evidence b(i)ased psychiatry. User-led research (Faulkner and Thomas 2002), carried out by 'experts by experience' in partnership with 'experts by study', focuses on issues and outcomes that are relevant to service users and does not pay 'blind' homage to the ultimate R(andomised) C(ontrol) T(rial) gold standard of scientific respectability. After all, it is the patients for whom these treatments are designed and in user-led research they can 'graduate' from passive subjects to equal partners (Trivedi & Wykes 2002). Yet, are there actually any research projects at all that have children and teenagers actively involved in designing truly meaningful searches for what works for whom? Furthermore, there is a publication bias in many 'respectable' journals, marginalizing or excluding research projects and papers that allegedly do not meet the (traditional) scientific criteria – and perhaps also do not fit with the dominant ethos and economic interests.

From context reading to context making

When visiting Child and Adolescent Mental Services up an down the country, no matter whether the are called 'Child Guidance', 'Child and Family Consultation' or 'Child and Adolescent Psychiatry', one tends to find in each clinic well established institutional practices. Children, teenagers and their families tend to get fairly similar assessments and treatments, no matter what their presentations, their problem history or their ethnicity. What is 'on offer' is said to be determined by the children's and families' perceived or postulated 'needs', as well as by the respective trainings and skills of the staff. These can vary enormously from clinic to clinic. The term 'need', so frequently used, if not misused, requires some discussion. Who actually defines 'need'? Do professionals identify certain 'needs' so that their interventions 'fit'? 'Need' is a social construction; it is not 'real' as such. It is therefore important to formulate jointly with families and referrers the treatment needs.

From a systemic perspective, when getting involved in any type of work, be that therapy, consultation, supervision or 'advice', clinicians on each occasion need to consider the context(s) within and out of which the request for 'help' arises. It can be helpful to think of doing this at different levels of the system: the level of the individual client, of the referrer, of significant others – including 'the family' –, at the level of culture and ethnicity, of the neighbourhood, the professional network, the political context and so on. This multi-level context reading can help clinicians with a systemic perspective to position themselves from the very outset. It allows them to consider at which level interventions can be made. Should we just work with the family? Do we need to involve the professionals / family network? How can we make use of the family's cultural connections to help the child with his problem? Should we see the child – or the parent – individually? When viewed from a systemic perspective, clinicians have plenty of choice, as there are many possible contexts within which the work can be carried out. Having read contextual issues, the next task is to make contexts that provide a response to the request for help. There is a basic question that can help clinicians to focus their work from the outset: 'what are the contexts that I need to use – or make – to address the presenting problems and issues?' In answering this question pragmatically, it is helpful to consider five types of 'context': there are different 'person contexts', a variety of 'time' and 'place' contexts, as well as a whole range of 'activity' and 'modality' contexts (Asen 2004).

The question of *who* ('person context') should be concretely present in a meeting or session opens up many possibilities – from partners to members of the extended family, from religious figures to neighbours, from other clinicians to politicians.

When considering *where* ('place context) the work is carried out there are usually a number of options: clinic setting, home, school, hospital ward, supermarket, court, mosque, community centre, town hall – the list would seem endless. Working with a child and family in a naturalistic setting, a setting where the problem manifests itself concretely, can be more effective than to confine all clinical work to sterile clinic settings or other agency-based interview rooms.

The 'time context' *(when?)* can be defined in terms of length, frequency and duration of the work. 10 or 20 minutes may be the appropriate time frame for carrying out preventive work in general practice, as this is the accepted 'time slot' and thus fits the primary care context. At the other end of the spectrum we have multi-problem families, with chronic histories and entrenched interactions with multiple agencies. They are not likely to make the required changes if they are at the receiving end of 60-minute sessions in fortnightly intervals. Here we may have to consider more realistic time frames and invent interventions that may last hours, maybe whole days, possibly with a frequency of four or five days a week – and a duration of two or three months, if not longer. Many of us were brought up with the '50 minutes hour', surely a time slot invented for the therapist's convenience rather than the client's. And if such therapy takes place five times a week for five years, is the time frame of this approach based on a careful reading of the client's specific needs and contexts – or is it a reflection of the therapist's 'prejudices', informed by a highly selective body of work? Whilst we allegedly enlightened clinicians may well smile at such seemingly old-fashioned psychoanalytic practices, are our practices actually all that different? Clinicians of whatever persuasion tend to create discreet time slots which then become institutionalised, lasting 60 or 90 minutes, with a 'magic' number of sessions (6 or 12) and some arbitrary duration of therapy (6 months or 1 year). The alternative to such predictable courses of clinical work would seem impracticable to many clinicians: anarchy and chaos might ensue if we tailor-made time frames for each child or family on each occasion. There are clinicians who argue that too much flexibility is confusing to our clients and others state that too much predictability and 'routines' is anti-therapeutic. Clinicians need to continuously think – and re-think – together with their clients whether the structures created or imposed (such as time) are still helpful. It is the joint process of continuous evaluation and revalidation of the clinical work that itself is healing.

What ('activity context') we do in our clinical work, the very 'activity', is clearly of major importance. Therapeutic work generally tends to be word-focused, with an ever-increasing preoccupation with 'narratives' and 'conversations'. This often marginalises children or excludes them altogether from what goes on in sessions. Yet, there are many non- or para-verbal ways undertaking clinical work, from ordinary play to psychodrama, from making collages to making music, from 'in vivo' exposure to 'real life issues' to staged multiple family events, from cultural encounters to working with local networks.

How ('modality context') clinicians do what they do, depends on their training, personal experiences and their 'self'. In the systemic field there are now plenty of diverse schools and orientations. All these approaches have developed at particular times and in highly specific contexts - as have other non-systemic approaches, be they psychodynamic, behavioural or somatic. It would seem limited and limiting to remain insecurely attached to just one 'religion' and proudly label oneself as a 'narrative' or 'structural' or 'solution focused' or 'post-Milan' therapist. Surely different presentations and problems, different cultural and social contexts, all would seem to require different responses from clinicians. Furthermore, the problems and preoccupations of our clients shift – we, the clinicians, also need to shift to keep up with our clients' movements. A therapeutic modality appropriate at the outset of clinical work may be second best only a few weeks later. If our therapeutic endeavours get stuck with a particular child or family, what use is it to do 'more of the same'? We talk about 'treatment resistant' patients and families – what about the change resisting clinician?

Using a systemic lens in clinical work opens up new perspectives and informs clinical practice. It helps to continuously question one's own work and practices and it leads to a flexible and innovative approach. The contextualising questions ('who?' 'where?' 'when?', 'what?' and 'how?') need not only be asked at the beginning of taking on new work, but throughout the whole process of clinical work with a child and family. By involving our clients in this questioning process we hopefully co-construct relevant contexts for change, opening up, for them and us, a multi-verse of new ways of seeing and experiencing. Systemic practitioners need to entertain multiple models simultaneously, systemic and non-systemic ones – if they want to contribute to generating multiple perspectives. The task of systemically oriented clinicians is then to manage, together with their clients, the multiple contexts that have been created to address the issues that led to the referral.

Context management

Adopting a systemic perspective permits clinicians to see the various different interventions in context and to construct maps for delivering complex simultaneous interventions in diverse contexts. Systemic clinicians are not only context readers and context makers – they are also natural context managers. For many of the more complex 'cases' referred to CAMHS, more than one intervention is likely to be made. Co-ordinating these different inputs are an important task, which avoids replication, contradictions and confusion. It requires a 'multi-modal' clinician, a professional who has the expertise and skills to provide multiple inputs at multiple levels and who is able to carry out and manage simultaneous work in different context. Instead of splitting children and families into different parts and farming them out to different professionals for different tasks and sub-tasks, possibly for the latter's convenience, multi-modal clinicians are able to integrate different models and approaches. Being systemic in orientation helps to have an overview and to provide an often necessary meta-perspective. It is an important step away from compartmentalised clinical practice which at present is 'owned' by various specialists – child psychiatrists, child psychologists, family therapists, child psychotherapists, CBT specialists, play therapists and so on.

Context managers are also able to carry out simultaneously both assessment and treatment functions, in the knowledge that all treatment contains aspects of assessment – and vice versa. Traditional child psychiatry teaches and preaches the virtues of undertaking so-called 'in-depth comprehensive assessments' of children and adolescents. This is an essentially medical approach, with the patients, be they children or adolescents – or occasionally adults – first having to subject themselves to a thorough examination. A battery of questions, questionnaires and tests can be levelled at the child and the carers. The main aim of this stage of the work is to make a diagnosis that informs the care plan. It is based on the traditional medical belief that one needs to know what 'it' is, so as to know how to treat 'it'. Whilst this is, at one level, a perfectly understandable quest, at another level children and families can be put off by lengthy or laborious assessment interviews. After all, parents and children usually attend a clinic to get some concrete help for their perceived problem(s) and not to be the subjects of some alien assessment procedure. Many families are seemingly compliant with such procedures, but then vote with their feet afterwards – particularly when they discover that therapeutic work is less valued in some academic centres.

Assessment does not have to be just a one-off snapshot of individual or family functioning. Assessment should also include the person's – or family's – ability to change. However, the ability to change can only be tested by putting in 'change inducing interventions' and this is where the distinction between assessment and treatment becomes blurred: assessment becomes also a therapeutic venture. The recursive process consists of clinicians observing what goes on, then commenting, then encouraging families to reflect and to identify new or different ways of doing things, trying it out and feeding back – to the clinicians – the outcome of their 'experiments'. Apart from making a diagnosis, the purpose of assessment is generally to ascertain whether changes can be made, in what timescale and whether they can be sustained. As a result, the time frames of assessments can be very varied, depending on the complexity of the task of change – it can be weeks or months.

Managing coinciding treatment and assessment contexts can be a complex task, particularly when working with families that have more than their fair share of problems, the so-called multi-problem or multi-crisis families. In these families, not generally courted by traditional child- and adolescent psychiatrists, because of their 'messiness' and their unwillingness to be fitted into neat diagnostic schemata, there are usually a number of members in simultaneous contact with different services: mental health, education and social services. Child abuse and neglect co-exist with domestic violence, drug and alcohol dependency, with school exclusion and delinquency. These families tend to be poor and disadvantaged and they are often subjected to racism and other forms of discrimination. When meeting these families, it is tempting to focus on family dysfunction and individual pathology. If, by contrast, one uses a family lens, then another focus emerges: instead of employing a deficit-based model, namely examining how families and their individual members have failed, it is possible to re-direct one's efforts to identifying of how families can succeed. Rather than writing off a seemingly 'hopeless' family's and attempting to rescue individual 'survivors' from its near-lethal grip, one can work with whole families and encourage their use of their own internal resources. The following case example hopefully illustrates the approach.

From multiple problems to multiple family work

Verna is a mother age 23, with 3 children under 5, each child with a different father, neither of whom is still around. Her current partner, Charlie, is the latest arrival on the family scene. He, like all the previous partners, is violent. Verna herself has had a horrendous history of physical and sexual abuse, emotional neglect, alcohol and drug abuse, a history of being in and out of foster and institutional care – as well as a history of being battered by all her partners. Social workers have always been in her life – and they still are now because of the serious concerns over the current welfare of Verna's children. There is no contact with her own family of origin and there are no lasting friendships – social workers appear to be the only stable and predictable presence in her life. It could be said that Social Services have become Verna's extended family.

When asked to assess Verna and her family, our team decided to see the family first in their own home – a very run-down council flat. Seeing families in their own homes allows much more naturalistic observation and understanding of how families live and function in their real life contexts. In Verna's home we saw plenty of family interaction, some good, some quite poor, some competent and some problematic parenting. When discovering that there were some twenty-three professionals involved with the family, our team speculated about the cycle of interaction between the family and the outside world. Such a high number of (more or less) involved professionals is not all that rare: multi-problem families usually turn into multi-agency families, as the anxieties these families evoke can often not be contained by a single or a few professionals alone. With each new crisis another opinion is sought, leading over time to a proliferation of professional input. It is commonly the case that the more workers become involved, the more potential for different opinions. And worse, the more external resources are made available to the family, the less confidence is there in the internal resources of the family. It was only a question of time until Verna herself felt totally disqualified as a person and as a mother, unable to think that she herself could offer anything useful to her children, let alone to anybody else.

When considering how to assess and intervene with Verna and her family, we were clear that she did not need more professionals in her system. However, we also knew that the existing professionals could not merely be 'fired' – they had become part of the system for a 'good' reason. If they left the field they would need to be replaced by someone else, otherwise Verna and her children would find themselves without a (professional) family. It is here that the setting of a 'family day unit' (Asen et al 1982, Cooklin et al. 1983) can be of great help. Such a place permits 6 – 8 families with similar issues and problems to attend together – for whole days and weeks. Not all families start and finish at the same time, as some may require less intensive work than others. The concept of a day unit for families is in line with the idea of connecting socially isolated parents and their families with one another. It is a 'living' context in which parents and families can contribute constructively to the welfare of other families and support each other during the stressful periods when they are attempting to achieve changes. Families receive feedback from other families attending the unit, providing opportunities to give constructive advice to one another and thereby feel validated in a helper- rather than patient-role. A level of emotional intensity, a 'hot house effect' can be achieved which is not usually possible in out-patient settings, bringing out the problems in relationships experienced within any given family in a dramatic fashion, but under relatively controlled and therefore safe conditions. A structured multi-family setting heats up family interactions and dynamics, families get 'cooked' or 'fried' much more quickly, displaying their familiar crises and thus permitting concrete resolutions of these. As a result, specific barriers to change, which constrain many of these families, are broken. A tightly constructed programme involves family members in interactional events of a great variety, e.g. as a couple, a family, as mothers with children, children by themselves, as individual adults, and so on. Different activities, such as outings, shopping trips, the joint preparation and eating of meals, or supervision of children's at times dangerous play, all make heavy demands on parents. Observing – and intervening in – conflict ridden family interactions and having problematic behaviours enacted 'live', makes it possible to understand how sequences arise and to test the potential for change 'in vivo'.

Verna and her three children attended our family day unit for 3 months and some of the work took also place in her home. She proved a very resourceful person – both in relation to her own family but also in relation to the five other families in the unit. She made friends with one family in particular and this was the beginning of her connecting with peers and disconnecting from the professional system. It took another 6 months of low intensity work in our unit and a lot of effort on her part to continue and sustain the changes. Follow-up a year later showed that the children were thriving in her care. She had sacked her boy friend and did not replace him with another one. She said that men were dispensable but her children were not. A few years later Verna came to our clinic for a social visit. She said that she had started a 'problem family support group' in the community centre near her housing estate – helping other families. She had also sent two of her friends and their children to our family day unit "so that they can learn what I learned". We now invite her, a past service user, from time to time to speak to other families, to tell her remarkable story of resilience, and how she overcame life's challenges.

Concluding recommendations and visions

Children and adolescents are almost always part of families and this is why it makes a lot of sense to see them in a family context. Parents usually have huge expertise even if this is often not all evident. Clinicians need to be continuously on the lookout as to how to make and create relevant contexts that bring out the resourcefulness in families and help them to help themselves. The expertise of CAMHS professionals needs to shift from clinic-based medically inspired practice to home- and community-based interventions, enabling families to connect with other families, rather than remaining over-connected with the helping system. This requires courage and innovative practices, including multiple service-user involvement, not as a politically imposed tokenism but as lived practice. Experts can be de-bunked when families become consultants to other families. Multiple family work, involving

6 – 8 families sharing similar problems, should be standard practice in clinics as well as in schools and other settings. In this model there is still a role for CAMHS clinicians, in the form of multi-modal workers, thus avoiding multiplication of helpers, as they are able – for a confined time – to deliver all the required interventions. Therapeutic intervention should begin during the first encounter between family and clinician, as part of what might be termed a 'therapeutic assessment'. The related-activities of context reading, context making and context managing should become essential skills that every CAMHS clinician is required to possess. And, last but not least, healthy irreverence towards any dogma, including the systemic one, is a prerequisite for good clinical practice and for respectful work with children, teenagers and their families.

References

Ackerman, N.W. (1967) *Treating the Troubled Family.* New York: Basic Books.

Andersen, T. (1987) The reflecting team. *Family Process* 26, 415 – 428.

Anderson, C.M. (1983) A psychoeducational program for families of patients with schizophrenia. In, W.R. McFarlane (ed.) *Family Therapy in Schizophrenia.* New York: Guildford.

Anderson, H., Goolishian, H.A. and Windermand (1986) Problem determined systems: toward transformation in family therapy. *Journal of Strategic and Family Therapy* 4, 1-13.

Asen, K.E., Stein, R., Stevens, A., McHugh, B., Greenwood, J. and Cooklin, A. (1982): A day unit for families. *Journal of Family Therapy* 4, 345-358.

Asen, E., Dawson, N. and McHugh, B. (2001) *Multiple Family Therapy. The Marlboroguh Model and its Wider Applications.* London & New York: Karnac.

Asen, E. (2004) Collaborating in promiscuous swamps – the systemic practitioner as context chameleon? *Journal of Family Therapy* 26, 280-285.

Bateson, G., Jackson, D., Haley, J. and Weakland, J. (1956) Toward a theory of schizophrenia. *Behavioural Science* 1, 251-264.

Cecchin, G. (1987) Hypothesising, circularity and neutrality revisited: an invitation to curiosity. *Family Process* 26, 405-13.

Cooklin, A., Miller, A. and McHugh, B. (1983) An institution for change: developing a family day unit. *Family Process* 22,453-468.

De Shazer, S. (1985) *Keys to Solutions in Brief Therapy.* New York: W.W. Norton.

Faulkner, A. and Thomas, P. (2002) User-led research and evidence-based medicine. *British Journal of Psychiatry* 180, 1-3.

Flaskas, C. (2002) *Family Therapy Beyond Postmodernism.* Hove and New York: Brunner-Routledge.

Foucault, M. (1975): *The Archaeology of Knowledge.* London: Tavistock.

Gergen, K.J. (1994): *Realities and Relationships: Soundings in Social Construction.* Cambridge, MA: Harvard University Press.

Goolishian, H. and Anderson, H. (1987): Language systems and therapy: an evolving idea. *Psychotherapy* 24, 529 – 38.

Haley, J.(1963) *Strategies of Psychotherapy.* New York: Gruner and Stratton.

Haley, J. (1979) *Leaving Home: Therapy for Disturbed Young People.* San Francisco: Jossey Bass.

Jones, E. (1993) *Family Systems Therapy: Developments in the Milan-Systemic Therapies.* Chichester: John Wiley & Sons.

Kuipers, L., Leff, J. and Lam, D. (1992) *Family Work for Schizophrenia: A Practical Guide.* London: Gaskell.

Laing, R.D. & Esterson, A. (1964) *Sanity, Madness and the Family*. London: Tavistock.

Leff, J., Kuipers, E., Berkowitz, R., Eberleinfries, R. and Sturgeon, D. (1982) A controlled trial of social intervention in schizophrenic families. *British Journal of Psychiatry* 141, 121-134.

Minuchin, S., Montalvo, B., Guerney, B.G., Rosman, B.L. and Schumer, F. (1967) *Families of the Slums*. New York: Basic Books.

Minuchin, S. (1974) *Families and Family Therapy*. London: Tavistock.

Minuchin, S. and Fishman, H.C. (1981) *Family Therapy Techniques*. Cambridge Mass.: Harvard University Press.

Sackett, D.L., Rosenberg, W.M.C., Gray, M., Haynes, R.B. and Richardson, W.S. (1996) Evidence based medicine: what it is and what it isn't. *British Medical Journal* 312, 71-72.

Selvini Palazzoli, M., Boscolo, L., Cecchin, G. and Prata, G. (1978) *Paradox and Counterparadox: A new Model in the Therapy of the Family in Schizophrenic Transaction*. New York: Jason Aronson.

Selvini Palazzoli, M., Boscolo, L., Cecchin, G. and Prata, G. (1980) Hypothesizing-circularity-neutrality; three guidelines for the conductor of the session. *Family Process* 19, 3-12.

Trivedi, P. and Wykes, T. (2002) From passive subjects to equal partners: qualitative review of user involvement in research. *British Journal of Psychiatry* 181, 468 – 472.

Vaughn, C. and Leff, J. (1976) The measurement of expressed emotion in the families of psychiatric patients. *British Journal of Social and Clinical Psychology* 15, 157 – 165.

Watzlawick, P., Jackson, D. and Beavin, J. (1967): *Pragmatics of Human Communication*. New York: W.W. Norton.

Watzlawick, P., Weakland, J. and Fisch, R. (1974) *Change: Principles of Problem Formation and Problem Resolution* New York: W.W. Norton.

White, M. and Epston, D. (1990) *Narrative Means to Therapeutic Ends*. New York: W.W. Norton.

9

The politics of Attention Deficit Hyperactivity Disorder (ADHD)

Sami Timimi

Introduction

A primary school struggling with being under-resourced, using labour intensive 'modern' educational methods in highly stimulating colourful classes, under pressure to demonstrate ever improving academic achievement in their pupils and with ever less acceptable methods for behavioural control of children at their disposal, finds out that John, One of their more distractible and boisterous children, has been given a diagnosis of ADHD and has started taking Ritalin. He is no longer as big a problem as he used to be; he does as he is told. The teachers now realize that John had a medical disorder and now that it's being treated he's not too bad. John's teacher also realizes that John's friend Paul seems to be similarly distractible and boisterous. She meets with Paul's parents and tells them that she wonders if Paul too has this 'ADHD' and advises them to see their general practitioner. Paul gets a diagnosis and starts taking Ritalin too. Soon other teachers in this school have started identifying children in their classes like John and Paul. A process has been set rolling. A year down the line John's old pattern of behaviour seems to be returning. Teachers agree that there could be many reasons for this (his parents have split up recently and he's started with a new teacher) but also wonder if it could be due to the treatment for his medical condition (ADHD) not being adequate. The school writes a letter that John's mum takes to his consultant and John's dose of Ritalin is increased. Soon Paul's dose also goes up. Other teachers talk about this and become aware that some of the children in their class may not be getting adequate medication. Another process is set in motion.

Meanwhile John's consultant has attended a couple of drug company sponsored seminars, has been contacted by a drug company representative and has been given parent and teacher information booklets by this representative (which describes ADHD as being caused by an inherited chemical imbalance in the brain and has pretty pictures of nerve cell synapses to show what's going-on in 'ADHD brains'). This literature now goes into local circulation and other parents' start contacting their doctor expressing concern that their child may have ADHD. A local parents' support group is set up and they join a national consumer pressure group (who organize yearly conferences with drug company financial help). The local paper interviews the parents' group who in turn talk about 'hidden disabilities' and how for years they struggled but no one recognized the psychiatric problem their children had. By now ADHD is firmly established in local culture with economically and politically powerful groups (drug companies, doctors and teachers) having had a major, but often unacknowledged, impact on a local community's conception concerning the nature of childhood. A new category of childhood has emerged- that of the ADHD child.

Something strange has been happening to children in Western society in the past couple of decades. The diagnosis of attention deficit hyperactivity disorder (ADHD) has reached epidemic proportions, particularly amongst boys in North America. In this country a child psychiatrist or paediatrician usually makes the diagnosis with advocates of the diagnosis claiming that children who present with what the diagnoser considers to be over-activity, poor concentration, and impulsivity are suffering from a medical condition, which needs treatment with medication. The main medications used for children with a diagnosis of ADHD are stimulants such as Ritalin, whose chemical properties are virtually indistinguishable from the street drugs speed and cocaine. Boys are four to ten times more likely to receive the diagnosis and stimulants than girls with children as young as two being diagnosed and prescribed stimulants in increasing numbers (Zito et al, 2000). By 1996 over six percent of school aged boys in America were taking stimulant medication (Olfson et al, 2002) with more recent surveys showing that in some schools in the United States over seventeen percent of boys have the diagnosis and are taking stimulant medication (Le Fever et al, 1999). In the UK prescriptions for stimulants have increased from 6,000 in 1994 to over 150,000 by 1999 (Department of Health, 1999), over a quarter of a million by 2002 (BBC news, 24th July, 2003), with the most recent figures showing that about 345,000 children in the UK were taking prescribed stimulants in the latter half of 2003 (Wright, 2003), suggesting that we in the UK are rapidly catching up with the US. Concerned professionals and parents are increasingly vocal in their criticism of the excessive use of stimulants.

In a failed attempt to silence its critics, ADHD advocates published an extraordinary consensus statement (Barkley et al, 2002) in which the most prominent professionals in this field accuse those who raise questions about the science and ethics of ADHD diagnosis and medication use, of being unscientific, "*To publish stories that ADHD is a fictitious disorder or merely a conflict between today's Huckleberry Finns and their caregivers is tantamount to declaring the earth is flat, the laws of gravity debatable, and the periodic table in chemistry a fraud*" (Barkley et al, 2002: 90). Most of authors of the statement are well known to have financial links with the pharmaceutical industry (which they do not declare in their statement) and it is no surprise that they conclude (despite the alarming rise in the amounts of stimulants being prescribed) that *"studies indicate that less than half of those with the disorder are receiving treatment"* (Barkley et al, 2002: 90).

The evidence is becoming clearer all the time and it does not make comfortable reading for the ADHD advocates. If the evidence in favour of conceptualizing ADHD as a neurological or neuro-developmental condition were already that good, then no statement would have been needed (Timimi et al, 2004). The ghost of nine eleven hides behind the tone adopted by their statement. Although the advocates have long dismissed their critics, nine eleven has seeped into the Western collective cultural unconscious and gives licence to those who wish to kill proper enquiry and debate through use of power and the 'You're either with us or against us' mind set.

A brief history of ADHD

Overactivity, poor concentration and impulsivity in children were first conceptualised as a medical phenomena earlier this century. The first recorded interest in children with poor attention and hyperactivity dates back to the turn of the last century when a paediatrician, Frederick Still, described a group of children who showed an abnormal incapacity for sustained attention, restlessness and fidgetiness, and went on to argue that these children had deficiencies in volitional inhibition, but offered no treatment other than good discipline (Still, 1902).

Hyperactivity and poor attention in children then came to be viewed as linked when the diagnosis of minimal brain damage (MBD) was coined. The idea of MBD had originally gained favour following epidemics of encephalitis in the first decades of the 20th century. Post encephalitic children often presented with restlessness, personality changes and learning difficulties. Then, in the 1930's, came a chance discovery that psycho-stimulant medication could reduce the restlessness, hyperactivity and behavioural problems that these children presented with (Bradley, 1937). Bradley believed that this calming effect he observed was likely to apply to anyone who took low dose stimulants, not just the hyperactive kids he was treating.

Not long after this episode, a number of doctors began to speculate that children who presented as hyperactive might have organic lesions in the brain that was causing their hyperactivity. Strauss's writings in the nineteen forties (e.g. Strauss and Lehtinen, 1947) strengthened this idea further by his suggestion that hyperactivity, in the absence of a family history of sub-normality, should be considered as sufficient evidence for a diagnosis of brain damage, believing that the damage was too minimal to be easily found.

By the nineteen sixties, however, the term MBD was losing favour as evidence for underlying organic lesions in children who displayed poor attention and over-activity was not being found. Instead, with the growing interest in behaviourally defined syndromes, the goal posts were moved and a behaviourally defined syndrome was articulated. Despite the abandonment of the minimal brain damage hypothesis the assumption that this syndrome does indeed have a specific and discoverable physical cause, related to some sort of brain dysfunction, survived in the new definition. Yet, studies have shown that demonstrable minimal brain damage due to a variety of causes, predisposes a child to the development of a wide range of psychiatric diagnosis as opposed to a particular type, such as ADHD (Schmidt et al, 1987). Rutter (1982) concluded that the available evidence shows that over-activity is usually not a sign of brain damage and that brain damage does not usually lead to over-activity. I am not aware of any research that contradicts that conclusion.

So it was that in the mid sixties the North American based Diagnostic Statistical Manual (DSM), second edition (DSM-II) coined the label 'Hyperkinetic reaction of childhood', to replace the diagnosis of MBD (American Psychiatric Association, 1966). Over the following three decades this new behaviourally defined condition rose from a matter of peripheral interest in child psychiatric practice and research in North America to a place of central prominence.

DSM II was replaced in the early eighties by the third edition (DSM-III, American Psychiatric Association, 1980). The disorder was now termed Attention Deficit Disorder (ADD). This could be diagnosed with or without hyperactivity and was defined using three dimensions (three separate lists of symptoms), one for attention deficits, one for impulsivity and one for hyperactivity. The three dimensional approach was abandoned in the late eighties when DSM III was revised (and became DSM-III-R, American Psychiatric Association, 1987), in favour of combining all the symptoms into one list (one dimension). The new term for the disorder was Attention Deficit Hyperactivity Disorder (ADHD), with attention, hyperactivity and impulsiveness now assumed to be part of one disorder with no distinctions. When the fourth edition of DSM (DSM-IV, American Psychiatric Association, 1994), reconsidered the diagnosis the criteria were again changed, this time in favour of a two-dimensional model with attention deficit being one sub category and hyperactivity-impulsivity the other. With each revision, a larger cohort of children is found to be above the threshold for diagnosis. For example, changing from DSM-III to DSM-III-R, more than doubled the number of children, from the same population diagnosed with the disorder (Lindgren et al, 1994). Changing from DSM-III-R to DSM-IV increased the prevalence by a further two thirds, with the criteria now having the potential to diagnose the vast majority of children with academic or behavioural problems in a school setting (Baumgaertel et al, 1995). Indeed according to DSM-IV, the diagnosis 'ADHD not otherwise specified' should be made if there are prominent symptoms of inattention or hyperactivity-impulsivity that do not meet the full ADHD criteria. If we were to interpret this concretely (as doctors often do) it suggests that nearly all children (particularly boys) at some time in their lives could meet one of the definitions and warrant a diagnosis of ADHD.

The modern champion of the ADHD diagnosis and one of the strongest advocates for a brain dysfunction model and the use of drugs to 'treat' these children is Professor Russell Barkley. Barkley's (1981) book *hyperactive Children: A Handbook for Diagnosis and Treatment*, received widespread attention from both the public and professional community. From there Barkley's campaign quickly caught the interest of the pharmaceutical industry and soon an avalanche of research to find more support for the disease theory and drug treatment ensued. Despite the volume of research and publications there is still no good evidence that supports the conclusion that ADHD is a medical disorder or that drug treatment is safe and effective (see below). DeGrandpre (1999) has aptly summarized the research that is being produced by the ADHD industry as 'junk science'.

ADHD, science or non-science (sense)?

So what is the evidence for the existence of this disorder? Is there a medical test that will diagnose it? No. Are there any specific cognitive, metabolic or neurological markers for ADHD? No. ADHD is a cultural construct diagnosed on the basis of clinical opinion and faithful belief of the practitioner and often presented as if it were a biological fact. Those who have argued that ADHD does not exist as a real disorder, start by pointing to the obvious uncertainty about its definition (McGuinness, 1989). Because of this uncertainty it is hardly surprising that epidemiological studies have produced very different prevalence rates for ADHD (in its various forms), ranging from about 0.5% of school age children to 26% of school age children (Taylor and Hemsley, 1995; Green et al, 1999).

There is a preponderance of boys over girls in ADHD symptomatology in the region of four (or more) to one (McGee et al, 1992). This is very similar to the gender distribution found in conduct disorder and other so-called externalising behavioural disorders in children. The meaning of this gender distribution is rarely questioned. What sort of biological variable are we attempting to categorise here if this is a biological abnormality? Is it that boys generally have bad genes compared to girls? Is it something to do with the normal biological differences between male and female genes? Is there an interaction between boy's behaviour and changes in social expectations regarding children's behaviour generally? Do social changes in family structure, lifestyles, teaching methods, classroom sizes, rates of violence, rates of substance misuse and so on have an effect on perceptions and beliefs about boy's and girl's behaviour, or even on their behaviour directly? Has life got harder for boys in some way? Has life got harder for parents trying to control normal boy behaviour? Are we still compelled to pay more attention to the externalised behaviour of boys than the internalised behaviour of girls, only now we medicalize this (after all adults in Western societies are usually more tolerant of hyperactivity in girls than in boys (Battle and Lacey, 1972))? Do changes in teaching methods have an effect on how we understand and deal with boys' behaviour? These and other social/cultural questions need to be discussed.

Despite attempts at standardising criteria and assessment tools in cross-cultural studies, major and significant differences between raters from different countries continue to be apparent (Mann et al, 1992). There are also significant differences between raters when raters rate children from different ethnic minority backgrounds (Sonuga-Barke et al, 1993). One replicated finding is an apparently high rate of hyperactivity in China and Hong Kong (Shen et al, 1985; Luk and Leung, 1989). In these studies nearly three times as many Chinese as English children were rated as hyperactive. A more detailed assessment of these results suggested that most of the 'hyperactive' Chinese children would not have been rated as hyperactive by most English raters and were a good deal less hyperactive than English children rated as 'hyperactive' (Taylor, 1994). One suggestion for such a consistently large disparity in hyperactivity ratings between Chinese and English children is that it may be due to the great importance of school success in Chinese culture leading to an intolerance of much lesser degrees of disruptive behaviour (Taylor, 1994). Whatever the reason(s), it demonstrates that hyperactivity and disruptiveness in boys is a highly culturally constructed entity.

That ratings of hyperactivity, inattention and disruptiveness are culturally dependent is not surprising as inattention, impulsivity and motor restlessness are found in all children (and adults) to some degree. Diagnosis is based on an assessment of what is felt to be developmentally inappropriate intensity, frequency and duration of the behaviours, rather than on its mere presence. All the symptoms described in this disorder are of a subjective nature (e.g. 'often does not seem to listen when spoken to') and therefore highly influenced by the raters cultural beliefs and perceptions about such behaviours. After all how do you operationalize, define and understand non-specific words like 'often' and 'excessive', which are invariably found in ADHD rating questionnaires?

What about co-morbidity? Numerous epidemiological and clinical studies demonstrate the high frequency with which supposedly separate child psychiatric disorders occur in individuals with ADHD (Caron and Rutter, 1991). In children with ADHD co-morbidity with other child psychiatric conditions is common no matter what definition is used (Beiderman et al, 1991). It is estimated that about half the children with ADHD also have a conduct disorder, about half also have an emotional disorder, about one third have an anxiety disorder and another third have depression (Barkley, 1994). Co-morbidity is so prevalent that at least three quarters of ADHD diagnosed children will have at least one other diagnosable child psychiatric condition (Hazell, 1997). The co-occurrence of the symptoms that make up oppositional/defiant and conduct disorders with those that make up hyperactivity and attention deficit disorders is so strong (Beiderman et al, 1991; Fergusson and Horwood, 1993) that many commentators have questioned the reality of the distinction between them. Psychiatrists have adopted co-morbidity as a way of trying to explain clinical reality when it does not appear to tally with research generated views of mental life. It's a way of maintaining a fantasy that there is a natural, probably biological, boundary where no natural boundaries exist (Tyrer, 1996).

This lack of a coherent concept is reflected in the lack of consensus on the question of possible causal mechanisms. Thus the condition was initially viewed as being due to an underlying, excessive motor activity in the child (Schachar, 1991) and later as being due to an underlying central attention deficit (Douglas, 1972; 1983). Others have suggested that the central deficit is one of generalised intellectual impairment (Werry et al, 1987) or of motivation (Draeger et al, 1986). The conviction held by a number of influential researchers about the likely central deficit has had a big influence on the behavioural definitions of the disorder. For example, Douglas's belief (1972) that attention, not hyperactivity, was the essential feature distinguishing these children from other difficult and disruptive children, led to the establishment of the 'Attention Deficit Disorder (ADD)' definition in DSM-III.

Claims have been made that neuroimaging studies confirm that ADHD is a brain disorder. Closer examination of the quoted studies not only reveals a more complex picture, it actually suggests the opposite, as the studies demonstrate that there is no characteristic neurophysiological or neuroanatomical pattern that can be found in children diagnosed as having ADHD. Brain scan studies have not uncovered a consistent deficit or abnormality, with a wide variety of brain structures being implicated, for example; Striatal, Orbital, Prefrontal, Fronto Posterior and Medial Orbital areas, Caudate Nucleus, Corpus Calosum and Parietal lobe (Rapport, 1995). The sample sizes in these studies have all been small and in no study have the brains of the ADHD diagnosed children been considered to be clinically abnormal (Hynd and Hooper, 1995), nor has any specific abnormality been convincingly demonstrated (Baumeister and Hawkins, 2001). Interestingly, after almost twenty five years and over thirty such studies, researchers have yet to do a simple comparison of unmedicated children diagnosed with ADHD with an age matched control group, the one large study that claimed to have done this (Castellanos et al, 2002) for reasons best known to themselves choosing a control group whose age was on average 2 years older (Leo and Cohen, 2003) and thereby all they scientifically managed to prove was that younger children had smaller brains than older ones! Most worryingly, animal studies suggest that any differences observed in these studies could well be due to the effects of medication that most children in these studies had taken (Breggin, 1999; 2001; Moll et al, 2001; Sproson et al., 2001).

What we end up with is speculative 'biobabble'. Even if consistent differences in neuro-imaging studies were found, unidirectional cause and effect cannot be assumed. This is because neurophysiological measures may reflect different children's different reaction to the same situation causing differences in brain chemistry rather than different brain chemistry causing different behaviour (Christie et al, 1995). Thus, differences in brain function have been demonstrated in normal healthy children who have different temperaments (Fox et al, 1995). At the turn of the century doctors used to measure the size and shape of the part of the skull housing the brain. They came up with all sorts of statistical differences and used these to justify a 'scientific' basis for amongst other things, the prevailing racist views of the time. This now discredited 'science', which lasted for over a hundred years before dying out early last century, was known as phrenology. It was believed that a skilled phrenologist could assess the moral and intellectual qualities of an individual by inspecting the skull and palpating its surface for characteristic bumps and protuberances. If we cannot stop ourselves from impulsively jumping to unwarranted conclusions about the reasons for differences found in brain scanning studies, we will create a modern version of phrenology.

In the rest of medicine, what has made diagnosis a useful way of categorising health problems, is that the diagnoses point to unique aetiological process (Beiderman et al, 1991; Klein and Riso, 1994; Taylor, 1988). In ADHD no unique aetiological processes have been identified, very much the reverse in fact as the evidence above demonstrates. Indeed, the National Institute of Health, a government body in the United States, concluded that there is no evidence to support the proposition that ADHD is a biological brain disorder (National Institutes of Health, 1998). This conclusion is further supported by a large body of family, twin and adoption studies that support the idea that a genetic component contributes to hyperactivity, conduct disorder and other externalising behaviours in a manner that suggests a common genetic mechanism underlies all these disorders (Timimi, 2002; Silberg et al, 1996). Presumably this common genetic mechanism has something to do with being a boy. As with neuro-imaging as soon as ADHD supporters focus on specifics, their argument starts to fall apart. Thus Schachar and Tannock (2002) argue that molecular genetic variations have been robustly replicated, concluding that ADHD is associated with the dopamine transporter gene (DAT1) and the dopamine receptor gene (D4); yet a recent study of 126 sibling pairs concluded that these two genes if they are involved in ADHD aetiology at all, make only a minor contribution to overall genetic susceptibility (Fisher et al, 2002).

If we take our starting assumption that behaviours such as motor activity, attention and impulsivity are normally distributed temperamental characteristics, then the evidence fits. Viewing these behaviours as temperamental characteristics as opposed to signs of a medical condition, allows more attention to context.

Research on children's temperament has shown that problems result from a mismatch between the child's temperament and their environment (Thomas and Chess, 1977; Chess and Thomas, 1996). Even children who are highly difficult temperamentally can become well adjusted behaviourally if their family and other social circumstances are supportive (Mazaide, 1989). What the genetic studies have been discovering is that the behaviours we call ADHD are probably inherited in much the same way as other personality traits, whether these behaviours come to be perceived as a problem is mediated by psychosocial factors.

Despite the overwhelming evidence that ADHD cannot be conceptualised in a simplistic, linear uni-causal way, authors in influential journals still write completely unsupported statements such as *"attention deficit hyperactivity disorder is a condition of brain dysfunction . . . it is a genetic, inherited condition"* (Kewley, 1998: 1594). Articles such as this that routinely appear in both medical and popular media and which offer an opinion masquerading as fact, contribute to the process of the ADHD construct being passed on from the medical profession to the general public and into general cultural consciousness as if ADHD were an already understood biological condition.

ADHD as culture specific solution to culture specific problems:

Thus far I have explored the history behind the development of the ADHD construct and the paucity of evidence to support the notion that ADHD is a neurological problem. Much of the inference thus far has been that the increasing use of the diagnosis of ADHD reflects a change in the meaning we give to childhood problems. But, it may also be true that there has been a real increase in ADHD type behaviours in children because of cultural, political, social and/or other environmental changes that have occurred in Western countries in the past few decades.

Life got tougher for American families. From the mid to late 1970's, a marked shift in social welfare policies took place. American businesses became less profitable and so began cutting wages, speeding up production, increasing automation, weakening unions and curtailing welfare programmes. Efforts were made to lower taxes to boost businesses resulting in re-distributing income upwards by providing tax cuts for those in the highest income brackets. Losses in government revenues were partly offset by cuts in social welfare programmes (Harvey, 1990; Phillips, 1990). The gap between rich and poor increased, with families bearing the brunt of the worsening social conditions.

Being a parent in North America has become more and more difficult. Issues such as violence, poverty and the breakdown of the family unit have been affecting ever-increasing numbers of families (Long, 1996). The index for the social health of the United States, which is produced by Fordham

University's Institute for social Policy, is based on 16 measures including infant mortality, homicide, teenage suicide, unemployment and drug abuse (Miringoff, 1994). This index gives a score ranging from 0 to 100 (with 100 being best). This index has declined from 74 in 1970 to 41 in 1992 indicating growing adversity facing US families. In 1994, there were over 4000 children murdered, over 15 million children living in poverty and over 14 million children living in single-parent families (Children's Defence fund, 1995).

At the same time as successive American governments were introducing policies to favour the business sector at the expense of a welfare safety net, an ideological shift was taking place in order to justify these actions. Social programmes were no longer viewed as humane or necessary, but as a potentially counter-productive effort that causes dependence and indolence amongst its recipients. An increased hostility developed toward the notion of dependence on the state, creating a new marginalized 'under-class', crowded into no-go urban areas where underground economies (such as the drug trade) developed (Cohen, 1997).

American right wing policies of a similar nature were imported into the UK in the early 1980's by the then British Prime Minister, Margaret Thatcher. The sense of social breakdown in the lives of children in this country (the UK) is also evident in recurrent media reports and debates about school crises, discipline problems, expulsion, violence in the young, crime in the young, bullying, drug abuse, break up of the family and breakdown in parent-teacher relationships. Psychosocial disorders amongst the young (such as suicide attempts, alcohol and drug abuse, and criminality) have shown a sudden and sharp rise throughout Europe and North America over the last couple of decades of the twentieth century (British Medical Journal, 1995). In the United Kingdom this has been occurring within the context of a dramatic widening of the social inequality gap with by far the biggest group effected being lower income families with children (Bradshaw, 1990).

Changes in social and political and economic circumstances are intimately connected with our common cultural beliefs and values. The last couple of decades of the twentieth century saw North America lead the way in promoting masculine competitive free market ideology and placing this at the centre of our value system. The end of the cold war has given capitalist free market ideology a sense of triumph, leading to 'socialism' becoming a bad word (abandoned even by the traditionally socialist British labour party). Dependence and nurture have come to be viewed as promoting passive helpless individuals who are of no use to society, and so the cult of competitive individualism has blossomed.

The knock on effect for children and families of this right wing capitalist ideology has been appalling. These social stressors are likely to have contributed enormously to the sadly negative experiences so many children in the West experience from the moment they are born. Children are growing up in families with no fathers, looked after by mothers who have no support networks and whom the state believes should be working (there is no esteem or importance attached to the work of a mother in Western society), in communities where drugs are sold at their school gates and rival gangs shoot at each other in next door flats. In a culture where children get in the way of heavily promoted individualistic desires of adults, parents of even middle and upper class children spend less and less time with their kids leaving a generation of children who feel abandoned and for whom 'home alone' has become a way of life (Kincheloe, 1998). Schools have to compete and boys who 'fail' academically (and it's mainly boys who do so in current school curricula) respond by building new identities (that reflect the dominant themes of individualistic capitalist ideology) around hyper-masculine notions such as fighting, football and fucking (Mac An Ghaill, 1994).

Could these increased life stressors for the young cause an increase in ADHD behaviours such as impulsivity, hyperactivity and distractibility? Perry and his co-workers (1995), pursuing a neuro-biological approach note how the symptoms of ADD/ADHD closely parallel those that occur during trauma- the hyper-alertness, the need to act quickly, the need to be on the go at all times in the expectation of danger and the inability to turn attention to matters other than those of physical safety. Their hypothesis is that, in a critical period in infancy some children experience trauma, which initiates a habitual automatic response, as though to some external threat. When older such children are sensitive to threat to a much greater extent than other children are and revert, as it were, to a state of 'red alert' very easily. Thus as with trauma induced stress, such children react quickly, over-actively, and not so much to their ordinary life as to anticipated threat.

Other 'brain development' researchers agree with this idea as more evidence is accumulating that shows that experience has physical effects on the developing brain which is now seen as an organ capable of undergoing reorganization in response to experiences, particularly in childhood but right up into adulthood (Valenstein, 1998; Bloom et al, 2001). Empirical support for this idea can be found in research on possible environmental causes of ADHD type behaviours that has been done which has found that psychosocial factors such as exposure to trauma and abuse can cause them (Ford et al, 1999; 2000; see chapter 5).

Breggin (1994; 1997) has put forward a strong case for the missing role of the absent father causing ADHD type behaviours and has renamed the syndrome DADD (Dad's Attention Deficit Disorder). He believes that loving attention from their fathers is an effective curative factor for these children. In a similar vein attachment theory suggests that the modern stressful social situations are having a dire and negative impact on the ability of parents to provide the sort of strong, secure and positive relationships children need with their parents. An accumulation of stresses on a family (such as lack of support, poverty, unresolved loss, poor relationship with father, insufficiently positive maternal model, pregnancy and birth complications), it is hypothesised, causes increasingly negative interactions to develop between a child and their parent(s) leading to exhaustion, frustration and irritability in the parent and challenging, hyperactive behaviour in the growing child, which in turn leads to a reinforcing demand-dissatisfaction cycle (Stiefel, 1997).

Lieberman and Pawl (1990), argue that impulsivity, recklessness, negative attention seeking, hyperactivity and poor concentration may represent a defensive adaptation on the part of a child in the context of such an insecure attachment relationship. Similarly, Speltz (1990) interprets the dyscontrol and non-compliance of young insecurely attached children as an attempt to control the proximity of the caregiver via problem behaviour. Putting the above hypotheses together- i.e. increased life stressors in modern society and the weakening of family structures leading to insecure attachment amongst children- we have a powerful culture specific explanation for an increase in ADHD type behaviours in the West. But there are plenty more.

A post-modern analysis of discourse and power, suggests that mother blaming maybe another important factor in the rise of ADHD diagnoses. In this explanatory model, mothers who hear the negative judgements of school and other parents, experience a profound sense of self-blame, failure, guilt and helplessness as well as anger and frustration at their child. When put in contact with the ADHD industry such a mother may, at least temporarily, feel freed from the mother-blaming context that has been so oppressive. She is no longer a failed mother, but a mother battling against the odds with a disabled child. In this analysis, the primary problem is not seen as residing in the mother or the child (or the often absent father), but in the effects of the dominant discourses of psychology, psychiatry and patriarchy, which render parent and child as passive and separated from their abilities, competence and strengths (Law, 1997).

Another culture specific set of ideas relates to our modern lifestyle. It is a common observation to note that whilst technology has given us all sorts of labour saving devices unavailable to earlier generation, we seem to have less time than ever. Our pace of life has been speeded up leading us to have higher expectations and a desire to 'do things', a desire that children absorb early in their lives. Various inventions have enabled us to live faster paced lives and have fed us higher levels of sensory stimulation, none more so than visual media like the television and computer. The increasingly centre stage role of electronic media that are fast paced, non linguistic, and visually distracting and that young children spend so many hours sat in front of, may literally have changed children's minds, making sustained attention to verbal input such as reading or listening, far less appealing than these faster paced stimuli. Exposure to TV and computer games from a young age could then lead to a form of sensory addiction and to problems when children are asked to adapt to more slow paced environments such as school (De Grandpre, 1999).

Interestingly, among the Amish, who are well known for their rejection of most modern indulgences such as computers and television, symptoms of ADHD appear to be uncommon (Papolos and Papolos, 1999).

Other modern lifestyle issues may also contribute to more ADHD type behaviours in our children. In the past, with parents having limited disposable income and there being fewer readily available sources of instant gratification, children had to learn through necessity to control their impulses. Nowadays, with instant gratification being such a big feature of the consumer culture, children are no longer being forced to learn early self-control of their impulses, a problem made worse by the belief that a diagnosis of ADHD means the child can't learn self-control (Timimi, 2002; 2005). Fears about children's safety, together with more 'in-house' entertainments such as computers and TV, have led to many children growing up with a lack of fresh air and exercise, leaving those more active boys to behave like 'caged animals' (Timimi, 2002; 2005). Junk diets, with excessive consumption of sweet foods and chemical additives, together with a lack of vital nutrients such as certain vitamins, minerals and amino acids has also been blamed for causing ADHD type behaviours (Hartmann, 1996).

Other theories relate to parenting. Life has become difficult for parents who are caught in a double pressure when it comes to discipline. On the one hand there are increased expectations for children to show restraint and self-control from an early age. On the other hand there is considerable social fear in parents generated by a culture of children's rights that often pathologises normal, well-intentioned parents' attempts to discipline their children. Parents are left fearing a visit from the SS (Social Services) and the whole area of discipline becomes loaded with anxiety. This argument holds equally true for schools. Parents often criticise schools for lack of discipline. Schools often criticise parents for lack of discipline. This double bind has resulted in more power going to children who are too young to handle it, thus breaking down their relationship to authority (Timimi, 2002; 2005). Furthermore, the task of parenting has come to be viewed as one that needs childcare experts' advice in order to get it right. A form of 'cognitive parenting' has arisen whereby parents are encouraged to give explanation and avoid conflicts (Diller, 2002). This hands-off, excessively verbal model of parenting is both more taxing and less congruent with children's more action based view of the world.

Other theories relate to changes in education. Schools are now expected to demonstrate better levels of academic achievement amongst their pupils and have to compete with other schools in national performance league tables. Much of the curriculum is being pushed 'downward' from older to younger children, with less time being set aside for more energetic and creative activities such as gym and music (Sax, 2000). Schools are arguably better set up for girl's development. Thus special needs support is four times more likely to be given to boys who lag behind girls in development of core school adaptive abilities such as reading and social skills. These two factors put together- more emphasis on academic achievement and differential rates of development- has put young-for-grade boys at a particular disadvantage resulting in as many as four fifths of young-for-grade boys being prescribed stimulant medication in some areas of North America (Le Fever et al, 1999; Ravenel, 2002).

The origins of the current epidemic of ADHD, lies deep in cultural machinery of Western society. There is less tolerance toward children (whose behaviour, particularly in boys, is thus more likely to be viewed as problematic) and a greater likelihood of medicalizing any perceived problem. At the same time it seems likely that we are seeing more ADHD type behaviours because of socio-cultural factors. Our (Western) cultural response to this problem is (not surprisingly) also culture specific and relates the powerful role of doctors in defining what meaning we give to everyday problems and of drug companies in using this medical invention as a powerful marketing tool.

The push toward greater use of the diagnosis and stimulants has been hugely influenced by the macroeconomics of drug company and doctors financial interests. In the US, with the managed healthcare system being the bread and butter of the majority of psychiatrists and paediatrician's work, when the more labour intensive psychotherapies lost favour with healthcare insurers, doctors soon realized they could make more money by going down the psychopharmacology route. Doctors can earn three times more by 15 minute medication review follow ups than a 45 minute visit with the child's family. Managed healthcare has meant that an economic system has come to be built around DSM IV diagnoses. In order to obtain a legitimate ticket to a service, you need a DSM IV diagnosis. Thus DSM IV has become more than a mental health diagnostic manual; it is a legal, financial and ideological document.

In the hierarchy of professional relationships, medicine is in a strong position to influence other professions also trying to deal with this growing anxiety about/hostility toward children. In America, behavioural psychologists, trusting that neurologists will, in time, discover the characteristics of the central nervous system that makes behavioural categorisations valid (Homans, 1993) took up the disorder and along with medical institutions passed the concept on to educationalists and eventually policy makers (United States Department of Education, 1991). Once greater cultural popularization of this concept occurred, children, particularly boys, who are either failing academically or exhibiting behavioural problems at home or at school, are suspected by a wide variety of professionals, parents, relatives and other influential people in the child's life, of having ADHD. The highly subjective nature of the DSM-IV definition allows for some very liberal interpretations, making ADHD well placed as a potential dumping ground for a whole host of problems. Wolraich et al (1990) showed that in only 30% of already diagnosed children in their study, did the home and school report both fulfil the DSM-IV diagnostic criteria.

The popularity of the ADHD diagnosis has been further strengthened through interest in the merits of prescribing stimulant medication to children. There is little doubt that in the short term 'methylphenidate', commonly known as 'Ritalin' (the stimulant most frequently prescribed to children), results in clinical improvement in many children who show hyperactivity and poor attention, with decreases in motor activity and defiance frequently reported (Greenhill, 1998). This observation has acted as a powerful reinforcer of the ADHD construct, many interpreting this as confirmatory evidence of the suspected physical causation (and therefore treatment) of the disorder. Baldessarini (1985) calls this sort of reasoning 'allopathic' logic, meaning that because a drug produces an effect, then there must be a disease. He sees this type of reasoning as false, misleading and invalid, after all we don't give Aspirin for a headache because headaches are caused by 'Aspirin deficiency'.

Stimulants central nervous systems effects are not limited to those children who can be defined by the boundaries of this disorder. Thus stimulants have the same cognitive and behavioural effects on otherwise normal children (Rapoport et al, 1978; 1980; Garber et al, 1996), aggressive children regardless of diagnosis (Spencer et al, 1996) and children with co-morbid conduct disorder (Taylor et al, 1987; Spencer et al, 1996). This is not surprising. The pharmacological action of Ritalin on the brain is basically that of amphetamines (or its street name – speed) and cocaine (Volkow et al, 1995), which is known to have similar effects in most people who take it.

Research has focused almost exclusively on short-term outcomes. Outcome research in Ritalin treatment has been shown to have serious shortfalls in methodology such as small samples, inadequate description of randomisation or blinding and not accounting for withdrawals or drop outs (Zwi et al, 2000; Joughin and Zwi, 1999). A recent meta-analysis of randomised controlled trials of methylphenidate found that the trials were of poor quality, there was strong evidence of publication bias, short term effects were inconsistent across different rating scales, side effects were frequent and problematic and long-term effects beyond 4 weeks of treatment were not demonstrated (Schachter et al, 2001).

The MTA group study (1999) has been highly influential and set a dangerous precedent in its conclusion that medication is better than psych-social therapies. This study has been widely criticised on many grounds, including lack of placebo group or blinding, authors being firm advocates of ADHD and well known recipients of drug company money, playing down of the numbers of children experiencing side-effects, participants already being 'cultured' into believing the children involved had a biological condition, study only lasting 14 months, and the fact that two thirds of those in the poorest outcome group (community treatment) were taking the very same stimulants. Some of the participants in the above study where followed up again after a further 10 months (in other words after a total of 24 months in the study). These results are not so impressive. While the percentages of children with normalized symptom levels (in other words those who in the opinion of the researchers were no longer displaying any ADHD symptoms) were essentially unchanged for the behaviour therapy only and community care groups, they had declined substantially for the combined (medication and behaviour therapy- from 68% to 47%) and medication only (i.e., from 56% to 37%) groups. The medication only group now had a similar percentage to the behaviour therapy only group. In addition, with regards social skills, reading achievement, and parents use of negative/ineffective discipline strategies there was no evidence of significant treatment group differences in the 24-month outcomes. Furthermore the children receiving medication were now significantly shorter than those who had not (MTA, 2004).

The few long-term studies that have been conducted suggest that stimulants do not result in any long-term improvement in either behavioural or academic achievement (Weis et al, 1975; Rie et al, 1976; Charles and Schain, 1981; Gadow, 1983; Hetchman et al, 1984; Klein and Mannuzza, 1991). Despite the lack of evidence for any long -term effectiveness, Ritalin is most usually prescribed continuously for seven, eight or more years, with children as young as two being prescribed the drug in increasing numbers despite the manufacturers licence stating that it should not be prescribed to children under six (Zito et al, 2000; Baldwin and Anderson, 2000).

The idea that Ritalin is a safe drug with few harmful side effects couldn't be further from the truth. Troublesome and frequently reported side effects include poor appetite, weight loss, growth suppression, insomnia, depression, irritability, confusion, mood swings, obsessive compulsive behaviours, psychosis, explosive violent behaviour, personality change, a flattening of the emotions which, when observed, looks like a zombie-like state, stomach ache, headaches, staring, disinterest, tachycardia, pituitary dysfunction and dizziness (Barkley et al, 1990; Breggin, 1999; 2002; Adrian, 2001). Cramond (1994) has also reported that treatment with Ritalin is associated with a lowered self-esteem and suppression of creativity in some children. Ritalin may also have long term adverse effects in as many as one third of those treated, including subtle cognitive effects such as perseveration (obsessive repetition of the same task), preoccupations, sombreness and deterioration in performance on complex cognitive tasks (Solanto and Wender, 1989; Sprague and Sleator, 1977). The lack of long-term studies into the effects of stimulants is a concern, as we do not really know what sort of effect giving an amphetamine like substance has on the developing brain.

Animal studies have found that taking stimulants can cause a long lasting change in the brain biochemistry of rats (Breggin, 1999; 2002; Moll et al,

2001; Sproson et al., 2001; Robinson and Kolb, 2001). We often forget that stimulants are powerful amphetamine like drugs with potentially addictive properties. Children become tolerant to its effect resulting in gradually increasing doses being given to children as years on a stimulant clock up. The potential for tolerance and addiction is further demonstrated by withdrawal states (known as the rebound effect, which manifests in increased excitability, activity, talkativeness, irritability and insomnia) seen when the last dose of the day is wearing off or when the drug is withdrawn suddenly (Zahn et al, 1980). Stories of adults becoming addicted to prescribed stimulants are becoming more prevalent (e.g. Wurtzel, 2002).

More difficult to assess is the possible socio-cultural effects such widespread use of stimulants in children may have. Doctors may be unwittingly convincing children to control and manage themselves using medication, a pattern that could carry on into adulthood as the preferred or only way to cope with life's stresses. Parents, teachers and others may lose interest in understanding the meaning behind an ADHD labelled child's behaviour beyond that of an illness internal to the child that needs medication.

In North America concern has been voiced about ADHD being diagnosed more frequently amongst children from families of low socio-economic status leading some authors to conclude that Ritalin is being misused as a drug for social control of children from disadvantaged communities (McGuinness, 1989; Kohn, 1989). The National Association for the Advancement of Coloured People in the United States has offered strong testimony that young blacks are over represented in the ADHD category and over medicated and has been campaigning for black parents to reject such a diagnosis (British Psychological Society, 1996). The dynamics of Ritalin prescription in North America have changed in recent years however, with the majority of those who get the prescription coming from white middle class families (Olfson et al, 2002). In this context one dynamic appears to be middle class parent's fears about their children's education. The anxiety is that that if their children don't get into college or university, they are 'sunk'. Thus parents and the middle class teachers of their children are converting this anxiety into requests for the perceived performance enhancing properties of stimulants and with more children in classrooms taking stimulants many parents end up feeling their child is at a disadvantage if they don't (Diller, 1998; 2002). This dynamic is reflected in the trend where stimulants are being prescribed to children without first making a diagnosis. This trend has now become so established that in some areas of the United States, less than half the children prescribed stimulants reach even the broad criteria for making a diagnosis of ADHD (Wasserman et al, 1999; Angold et al, 2000).

Ritalin is a drug of abuse as it can be crushed and snorted to produce a high (Heyman, 1994). Surveys have shown that a significant proportion of adolescents in the United States self report using Ritalin for non-medical purposes (Robin and Barkley, 1998). Accounts of abuse of Ritalin and other stimulants are increasingly being reported in the lay press (Ravenel, 2002). A national survey in the United States found that 2.8% of high school seniors had used Ritalin without a physician's prescription the previous year (Sannerud and Feussner, 2000). The neuro-chemical effects of Ritalin are very similar to that of Cocaine, which is one of the most addictive drugs. Cocaine users report that the effect of injected Ritalin is almost indistinguishable from that of Cocaine (Volkow et al, 1995). Biederman's (1999) study on the likelihood of substance misuse amongst those with a diagnosis of ADHD treated with a stimulant concluded that they were less likely to abuse substances when compared to those with ADHD who were not treated with stimulants. However, a much larger, community based study (Lambert and Hartsough, 1998) found a significant increase in cocaine and tobacco dependence amongst ADHD subjects taking stimulants when compared to controls, furthermore they discovered a linear relationship between the amount of stimulant treatment and the likelihood of either tobacco or cocaine dependence.

Thus Ritalin remains a controversial drug for reasons that go well beyond its side effects. Yet these issues that should be important information for all parents trying to make the difficult decision as to whether or not to agree for their children to take a stimulant, is information that is rarely given by prescribers (Baldwin and Cooper, 2000)

The phenomenal rise in stimulant prescribing has led to the suggestion that ADHD has been conceived and promoted by the pharmaceutical industry in order for there to be an entity for which stimulants could be prescribed (McGuinness, 1989). It is after all a multi million dollar industry, with the National Institute of Mental Health (Karon, 1994), the US Department of Education and the Food and Drug Administration (Breggin, 1994) all having been involved in funding and promoting treatment which calls for medicating children with behavioural problems. It has been claimed that the pharmaceutical companies Ciba & Novartis conspired and colluded to develop and promote the diagnosis of ADHD in a highly successful effort to increase the market for its product, Ritalin. This effort has included funding parent support groups, pro-medication research and payments to professionals to act as spokespeople for their companies or products (Breggin, 2000). The situation with drug companies controlling the agenda of scientific debate has become so bad that it is virtually impossible to climb up the career ladder without promotional support (e.g. to fund research, to speak at conferences, to write papers for journals) from drug companies. Thus we have reached the situation were most senior academics have long standing financial links with drug companies, that inevitably seriously compromises the impartiality of their opinions (Burton and Rowell, 2003). Similarly the impartiality of patient support organizations has to be questioned. In recent years it has become apparent that drug companies are using such consumer lobbying groups to their advantage not only by (often secretly) generous donations, but also on occasion by setting up patient groups themselves (Herxheimer, 2003). The main pro-medication pro-ADHD consumer support group in North America is CHADD, which receives substantial amounts from drug companies, receiving an estimated $500,000 in 2002 (O'Meara, 2003). There are other support groups, for example in the United Kingdom the parent support group 'Overload', have been campaigning for prescribing doctors to provide more information to parents about the cardiovascular and neurological side effects of stimulants, believing that many more parents would be likely to reject such medication if they were being properly informed about it by the medical profession. However, without the financial support of the multinational giants, their message rarely gets heard.

Conclusion: Developing non-toxic solutions for ADHD type behaviours:

As with non-medical theories of causation, non-drug-based solutions to the problems children with ADHD type behaviours present have been marginalized by the more politically powerful, Drug Company supported medical and consumer bodies. A comprehensive set of therapeutic strategies and approaches needs to be able to tackle the issues sited above, from the adverse effects of labelling, therapy with the child concerned right up to working with parents, schools and the local community. This does not mean doing all of these with all children referred but what it does mean is a wholesale shift in attitude away from that of labelling kids with a medical disorder, in the absence of any evidence that they are suffering from a physical defect.

In my opinion, the starting point for offering a holistic, integrated, multi-perspective model has to be the rejection of ADHD as label that offers anything meaningful or useful to clinical practice. Paradoxically, although the use of the ADHD diagnosis and stimulant medication may appear to offer a cheap, labour saving way of helping these children and their families, as with stimulants effectiveness it does the opposite. Although you may get quick results in the short term, in the long term you create a group of children who are dependent (on the drugs and the doctors who prescribe them) and need to carry on seeing their doctor for years (some say the rest of their lives), without ever having dealt with the original difficulties. My experience is that if I see my basic role as that of empowering children, parents and schools to find their own solutions, then dependency on doctors doesn't happen and my clients can be discharged from my clinics in a comparatively short time and with at least as good an outcome (particularly in terms of client's satisfaction) than going down the more labour intensive (in the long term) diagnosis and medication route.

In terms of what might be considered 'modernist' (expert derived) interventions useful approaches include family and systemic therapy, such as interventions to improve communication and relationships in the family, address attachment issues, explore family and parental history, and consult with schools and other professionals (e.g. Alexander and Parsons, 1982, Alexander et al, 1988, Henggeller and Borduin, 1990, Oas, 2001); specific behaviour management strategies, such as those to enforce effective discipline (e.g. Stein, 2001, Breggin, 2000, Sells, 2001); addressing lifestyle issues, such as slowing down the pace of life, creating more family time, regular opportunities for exercise and looking at diet (e.g. De Grandpre, 1999, Armstrong, 1995, Jacobson and Schardt, 1999); and a discussion of the families value system as well as a questioning of one's own cultural values and how this may effect practice (e.g. Timimi, 2003).

In terms of post-modern style interventions (privileging families existing knowledge), although little has been written specifically about ADHD, postmodern thinking has informed many useful therapeutic interventions including deconstructing traditional medical and psychological discourses (e.g. Law, 1997, Smith and Nylund, 1997); focusing on strengths and building solutions (e.g. Shazer, 1994); use of metaphor and stories (e.g. Rosen, 1982, Dwivedi, 1997), externalizing the problem (e.g. White and Epston, 1990, Smith and Nylund, 1997) and advocacy work on behalf of the family (Timimi, 2002). For the sake of convenience I have called the style of working that includes all these differing metaphors that we use in therapy to construct a (hopefully) meaningful and useful intervention a 'multi-perspective' approach (Timimi, 2002; 2005). Using this approach I have, in collaboration with their families, successfully weaned over 30 children off of stimulant medication in the past 2 years, without needing to start such a prescription for a single child, leaving me with no children on my current caseload that take a stimulant.

References

Adrian, N. (2001) Explosive outbursts associated with methylphenidate. *Journal of the American Academy of Child and Adolescent Psychiatry* 40, 618-619.

Alexander, J.F. and Parsons, B.V. (1982) *Functional family therapy.* Monterey, C.A.: Brooks-Cole.

Alexander, J.F., Waldron, H.B., Newberry, A.M. and Liddle, N. (1988) Family approaches to treating delinquents. In E.W. Nunnally, C.S. Chilman and F.M. Cox, (Eds) *Mental Illness, Delinquency, Addictions and Neglect.* Newbury Park, C.A.: Sage.

American and Psychiatric Association (1966) *Diagnostic Statistical Manual of Mental Disorders, Second Edition (DSM-II).* Washington DC: APA.

American and Psychiatric Association (1980) *Diagnostic Statistical Manual of Mental Disorders, Third Edition (DSM-III).* Washington DC: APA.

American Psychiatric Association (1987) *Diagnostic and Statistical Manual of Mental Disorders, Third Edition Revised (DSM-III-R).* Washington DC: APA.

American Psychiatric Association (1994) *Diagnostic and Statistical Manual of Mental Disorders, Fourth Edition (DSM-IV).* Washington DC: APA.

Angold, A., Erkanli, A., Egger, H.L. and Costello, E.J. (2000) Stimulant treatment for children: A community perspective. *Journal of the American Academy of Child and Adolescent Psychiatry* 39, 975-984.

Armstrong, T. (1995) *The Myth of the ADD Child.* New York: Dutton.

Baldessarini, R.J. (1985) *Chemotherapy in Psychiatry: Principles and Practice.* Cambridge, MA: Harvard University Press.

Baldwin, S. and Anderson, R. (2000) The cult of methylphenidate: Clinical update. *Critical Public Health* 10, 81-86.

Baldwin, S. and Cooper, P. (2000) How should ADHD be treated? *The Psychologist* 13, 598-602.

Barkley, R.A. (1981) *Hyperactive Children: A Handbook for Diagnosis and Treatment.* New York: Guilford Press.

Barkley, R.A. (1994) Attention Deficit Hyperactivity Disorder. *Presentation at the Royal Society of Medicine* London, 1994.

Barkley, R.A. et al (2002) International Consensus Statement on ADHD. *Clinical Child and Family Psychology Review* 5, 89- 111.

Barkley, R.A., McMurray, M.B., Edelbrock, C.S. and Robbins, K. (1990) Side-effects of methylphenidate in children with attention deficit hyperactivity disorder: a systematic, placebo-controlled evaluation. *Paediatrics* 86, 184-192.

Battle, E.S. and Lacey, B. (1972) A context for hyperactivity in children over time. *Child Development* 43, 757-773.

Baumeister, A.A. and Hawkins, M.F. (2001) Incoherence of neuroimaging studies in attention deficit/hyperactivity disorder. *Clinical Neuropharmacology,* 24, 2-10.

Baumgaertel, A., Wolraich, M.L. and Dietrich, M. (1995) Comparison of diagnostic criteria for Attention Deficit Disorders in a German elementary school sample.

Journal of the American Academy for Child and Adolescent Psychiatry 34, 629-638.

Biederman, J. (1999) Pharmacotherapy of attention deficit/hyperactivity disorder reduces the risk for substance use disorder. *Pediatrics.* 104: e20-e30.

Biederman, J., Newcorn, J. and Sprich, S. (1991) Comorbidity of attention deficit disorder with conduct, depressive, anxiety and other disorders. *American Journal of Psychiatry* 148, 564-577.

Bloom, F.E., Nelson, C.A. and Lazerson, A. (2001) *Brain, Mind and Behavior (Third Edition).* New York: Worth Publications.

Bradley, C. (1937) The behaviour of children receiving Benzedrine. *American Journal of Psychiatry* 94, 577-585.

Bradshaw, J. (1990) *Child Poverty and Deprivation in the United Kingdom.* London: National Children's Bureau.

Breggin, P. (1994) *The War Against Children: How the Drugs Programmes and Theories of the Psychiatric Establishment are Threatening America's Children with a Medical 'Cure' for Violence.* New York: St Martin's Press.

Breggin, P. (1997) *The Heart of Being Helpful: Empathy and the Creation of a Healing Presence.* New York: Springer Publishing Company.

Breggin, P. (1999) Psychostimulants in the treatment of children diagnosed with ADHD: Part II- Adverse effects on brain and behavior. *Ethical Human Sciences and services* 1, 213-241.

Breggin, P. (2000) The NIMH multimodal study of treatment for attention deficit/ hyperactivity disorder: A critical analysis. *International Journal of risk and safety in medicine* 13, 15-22.

Breggin, P. (2001a) *Talking Back to Ritalin: What Doctors Aren't Telling You about Stimulants for Children (revised edition).* Cambridge, MA: Perseus Publishing.

Breggin, P. (2002) *The Ritalin Fact Book.* Cambridge, MA: Perseus Publishing.

British Medical Journal News (1995) *British Medical Journal* 310, 1429.

British Psychological Society (1996) *Attention Deficit Hyperactivity Disorder (ADHD): A psychological response to an evolving concept, Report of a working party of the BPS.* London: British Psychological Society.

Burton, B. and Rowell, A. (2003) Unhealthy spin. *British Medical Journal.* 326: 1205-1207

Caron, C. and Rutter, M. (1991) Comorbidity in child psychopathology: concepts, issues and research strategies. *Journal of Child Psychology and Psychiatry* 32, 1063-1080.

Castellanos, F.X., Lee, P.P., Sharp, W., et al (2002) *Developmental Trajectories of Brain Volume Abnormalities in Children and Adolescents with Attention-Deficit/ Hyperactivity Disorder.* Journal of the American Medical Association, 288, 1740-1748

Charles, L. and Schain, R. (1981) A four year follow up study of the effects of methylphenidate on the behaviour and academic achievement of hyperactive children. *Journal of Abnormal Child Psychology* 9, 495-505.

Chess, S. and Thomas, A. (1996) *Temperament Theory and Practice*. New York: Brunner Mazel.

Children's Defence Fund (1994) *The State of America's Children Yearbook: 1994.* Washington D.C: Children's Defence Fund.

Christie, D., Lieper, A.D., Chessells, J.M. and Vergha-Khadem, F. (1995) Intellectual performance after presymptomatic cranial radiotherapy for leukaemia: effects of age and sex. *Archives of Disease in Childhood* 73, 136-140.

Cohen, C. (1997) The political and moral economy of mental health. *Psychiatric Services* 48, 768-774.

Cramond, B. (1994) Attention Deficit Hyperactivity Disorder and creativity: What is the connection? *Journal of Creative Behaviour* 28, 193-210.

De Grandpre, R. (1999) *Ritalin Nation*. New York: WW Norton.

Department of health (1999) *Prescription Cost Analysis*. London: Department of Health.

Diller, L.H. (1998) *Running on Ritalin*. New York: Bantam.

Diller, L.H. (2002) ADHD: real or an American myth. *Presented at the 14th Annual Conference of the Associazone Cultural Pediatri*. Rome: 10th of October 2002

Douglas, V.I. (1972) Stop, look and listen: the problems of sustained attention and impulse control in hyperactive and normal children. *Canadian Journal of Behavioural Science* 4, 254-282.

Douglas, V.I. (1983) Attention and cognitive problems. In M. Rutter (Ed) *Developmental Neuro-Psychiatry*. New York: Guildford.

Draeger, S., Prior, M. and Sanson, A. (1986) Visual and auditory attention performance in hyperactive children: competence or compliance. *Journal of Abnormal Child Psychology* 14, 411-424.

Dwivedi, K.N (1997) Management of anger and some Eastern stories. In K.N. Dwivedi (Ed) *Therapeutic Use of Stories*. London: Routledge.

Fergusson, D.M. and Horwood, L.J. (1993) The structure, stability and correlations of the trait components of conduct disorder, attention deficit disorder and anxiety withdrawal reports. *Journal of Child Psychology and Psychiatry* 34, 749-766.

Fisher, S.L., Francks, C., McCracken, J.T., et al. (2002). A genome-wide scan for loci involved in Attention Deficit/Hyperactivity Disorder (ADHD). *American Journal of Human Genetics*, 70, 1183-1196.

Ford, J.D., Racusin, R., Daviss, W.B., et al. (1999) Trauma exposure among children with oppositional defiant disorder and attention deficit-hyperactivity disorder. *Journal of consulting and Clinical Psychology* 67, 786-789.

Ford, J.D., Racusin, R., Ellis, C.G., Daviss, W.B., Reiser, J., Fleischer, A. and Thomas, J. (2000) Child maltreatment, other trauma exposure, and posttraumatic symptomatology among children with oppositional defiant and attention deficit hyperactivity disorders. *Child Maltreatment* 5, 205-217.

Fox, N.A., Rubin, K.H., Calkins, S.D., et al. (1995) Frontal activation asymmetry and social competence at four years of age. *Child Development* 66, 1770-1784.

Gadow, K.D. (1983) Effects of stimulant drugs on academic performances in hyperactivity and learning disabled children. *Journal of Learning Disabilities* 16, 290-299.

Garber, S.W., Garber, M.D. and Spizman, R.F. (1996) *Beyond Ritalin*. New York: Harper Perennial.

Green, M., Wong, M., Atkins, D., Taylor, J. and Feinleib, M. (1999) *Diagnosis of Attention Deficit Hyperactivity Disorder*. Rockville MA: Agency for Healthcare Policy and Research.

Greenhill, L. (1998) Childhood ADHD: Pharmacological treatments. In P. Nathan and J. Gorman (Eds.) *A Guide to Treatments that Work*. Oxford: Oxford University Press.

Hartman, T. (1996) Beyond *ADD: Hunting for reasons in the past and present*. Grass Valley, CA: Underwood Books.

Harvey, D. (1990) *The Condition of Postmodernity*. Oxford: Blackwell.

Hazell, P. (1997) The overlap of attention deficit hyperactivity disorder with other common mental disorders. *Journal of Paediatric Child Health* 33, 131-137.

Hengeller, S.W. and Borduin, C.M. (1990) *Family Therapy and Beyond: A Multi-Systemic Approach to Treating the Behaviour Problems of Children and Adolescents*. Pacific Grove, CA: Brooks-Cole.

Herxheimer, A. (2003) Relationships between pharmaceutical industry and patients organizations. *British Medical Journal* 326, 1208-1210.

Hetchman, L., Weis, G. and Perlman, T. (1984) Young adult outcome of hyperactive children who received long term stimulant medication. *Journal of the American Academy of Child and Adolescent Psychiatry* 23, 261-269.

Heyman, R. (1994) Methylphenidate (Ritalin): Newest drug of abuse in schools. *Ohio Paediatrics* spring, 17-18.

Homans, G.C. (1993) Behaviourism and after. In A. Giddens and J. Turner (Eds.) *Social Theory Today*. Cambridge: Polity Press.

Hynd, G.W. and Hooper, S.R. (1995) *Neurological Basis of Childhood Psychopathology*. London: Sage Publications.

Jacobson, M. and Schardt, D. (1999) *Diet, ADHD and Behavior: A Quarter-Century Review*. Washington: Center for Science in the Public Interest.

Joughin, C. and Zwi, M. (1999) *Focus on the Use of Stimulants in Children with Attention Deficit Hyperactivity Disorder. Primary Evidence-Base Briefing No.1*. London: Royal College of Psychiatrists Research Unit.

Karon, B.P. (1994) Problems of psychotherapy under managed care. *Psychotherapy in Private Practice* 2, 55-63.

Kewley, G.D. (1998) Attention Deficit Hyperactivity Disorder is under diagnosed and under treated in Britain. *British Medical Journal* 316, 1594-1595.

Kincheloe, J.L. (1998) The new childhood: Home alone as a way of life. In H. Jenkins (Ed.) *The Children's Culture Reader*. New York: New York University Press.

Klein, D.N. and Riso, L.P. (1994) Psychiatric disorders: problems of boundaries and comorbidity. In C.G. Costello (Ed.) *Basic Issues in Psychopathology*. New York: Guildford Press.

Klein, R.G. and Mannuzza, S. (1991) Long-term outcome of hyperactive children: A review. *Journal of American Academy of Child and Adolescent Psychiatry* 30, 383-387.

Kohn, A. (1989) Suffer the restless children. *Atlantic Monthly* Nov 90-100.

Lambert, N.M., and Hartsough, C.S. (1998) Prospective study of tobacco smoking and substance dependence among samples of ADHD and non-ADHD participants. *Journal of Learning Disabilities* 31, 533-544.

Law, I. (1997) Attention deficit disorder- therapy with a shoddily built construct. In C. Smith and D. Nyland (Eds.) *Narrative therapies with children and adolescents.* New York: The Guildford Press.

LeFever, G.B., Dawson, K.V., and Morrow, A.D. (1999) The extent of drug therapy for attention deficit hyperactivity disorder among children in public schools. *American Journal of Public Health* 89, 1359-1364.

Leo, J.L. and Cohen, D.A. (2003) Broken brains or flawed studies? A critical review of ADHD neuroimaging research. *The Journal of Mind and Behavior* 24, 29-56.

Lieberman, A.F. and Pawl, J.H. (1990) Disorders of attachment and secure base behaviour in the second year of life. In M.T. Greenberg, D. Cicchetti and E.M. Cummings (Eds.) *Attachment in the Preschool Years.* Chicago: University of Chicago Press.

Lindgren, S., Wolraich, M., Stromquist, A., Davis, C., Milich, R. and Watson, D. (1994) Reexamining Attention Deficit Disorder. *Presented at the 8th annual meeting of the Society for Behavioural Paediatrics,* Denver.

Long, N. (1996) Parenting in the USA: Growing adveristy. *Clinical Child Psychology and Psychiatry* 1, 496-483.

Luk, S.L. and Leung, P.W.L. (1989) Connors teachers rating scale – a validity study in Hong Kong. *Journal of Child Psychology and Psychiatry* 30, 785-794.

Mac An Ghaill, M. (1994) *The Making of Men: Masculinities, Sexualities and Schooling.* Buckingham: Open University Press.

Mann, E.M., Ikeda, Y., Mueller, C.W., Takahashi, A., Tao, K.T., Humris, E., Li, B.L. and Chin, D. (1992) Cross-cultural differences in rating hyperactive-disruptive behaviours in children. *American Journal of Psychiatry* 149, 1539-1542.

Mazaide, M. (1989) Should adverse temperament matter to the clinician? An empirically based answer. In G.A. Khonstaum, V.E. Bates and M.K. Rothbart (Eds.) *Temperament in Childhood.* New York: Wiley.

McGee, R., Feehan, M., Williams, S. and Anderson, J. (1992) DSM-III disorders from age 11 to age 15 years. *Journal of the American Academy for Child and Adolescent Psychiatry* 31, 50-59.

McGuiness, D. (1989) Attention Deficit Disorder, the Emperor's new clothes, Animal 'Pharm' and other fiction. In S. Fisher and R. Greenberg (Eds.) *The Limits of Biological Treatments for Psychological Distress: Comparisons with Psychotherapy and Placebo.* Hillsdale, N.J: Lawrence Erlbaum Associates

Miringolt, M. (1994) *Monitoring the Social Well-Being of the Nation: The Index of Social Health.* Tarytown, N.Y: Fordham Institute for Social Policy.

Moll, G., Hause, S., Ruther, E., Rothenberger, A. and Huether, G. (2001) Early methylphenidate administration to young rats causes a persistent reduction in the density of striatal dopamine transporters. *Journal of Child and Adolescent Psychopharmacology* 11, 15-24.

MTA Co-operative Group (1999) A 14 month randomized clinical trial of treatment strategies for attention deficit/hyperactivity disorder. *Archives of General Psychiatry* 56, 1073-1086.

MTA Co-operative Group (2004) National Institute of Mental Health Multimodal Treatment Study of ADHD follow-up: *24-month Outcomes of Treatment Strategies for Attention-Deficit/Hyperactivity Disorder.* Pediatrics 113, 754-761.

National Institutes of Health (1998) *Consensus Statement: Diagnosis and Treatment of Attention Deficit Hyperactivity Disorders.* Rockville, M.D: National Institute of Mental Health.

Oas, P. (2001) *Curing ADD/ADHD Children.* Raleigh, NC: Pentland Press.

Olfson, M., Marcus, S.C., Weissman, M.M. and Jensen, P.S. (2002) National trends in the use of psychotropic medications by children. *Journal of the American Academy of Child and Adolescent Psychiatry* 41, 514-21.

O'Meara, P. (2003) Putting power back in parental hands. *Insight Magazine* 28th April 2003.

Papolos, D. and Papolos, J. (1999) *The Bipolar Child.* New York: Broadway Books.

Perry, B.D., Pollard, R.A., Blackeley, T.L., Baker, W.L. and Vigilante, D. (1995) Childhood trauma, the neurobiology of adaptation and the use-dependent development of the brain, how states become traits. *Infant Mental Health Journal* 16, 20-33.

Phillips, K. (1990) *The Politics of Rich and Poor.* New York: Random House.

Rapoport, J.L., Buchsbaum, M.S., Zahn, T., Weingartner, H., Ludlow, C. and Mickkelsen, E.J. (1978) Dextroamphetamine: cognitive and behavioural effects in normal prepubertal boys. *Science* 199, 560-563.

Rapoport, J.L., Buchsbaum, M.S., Zahn, T., Weingarten, H., Ludlow, C. and Mickkelsen, E.J. (1980) Dextroamphetamine: Its cognitive and behavioural effect in normal and hyperactive boys and normal men. *Archives of General Psychiatry* 37, 933-943.

Rapport, M.D. (1995) Attention Deficit Hyperactivity Disorder. In M. Hersen and R.T. Ammerman (Eds.) *Advances in Abnormal Child Psychology.* Hillsdale, N.J: Lawrence Erlbaum Associates.

Ravenel, D.B. (2002) A new behavioral approach for ADD/ADHD and behavioral management without medication. *Ethical Human Sciences and Services* 4, 93-106.

Rie, H., Rie, E., Stewart, S. and Anbuel, J. (1976) Effects of Ritalin on underachieving children: A replication. *American Journal of Orthopsychiatry* 45, 313-332.

Robin, A.L. and Barkley, R.A. (1998) *ADHD in Adolescents: Diagnosis and Treatment.* New York: Guildford.

Robinson, T.E., and Kolb, B. (2001) Persistent structural modifications in nucleus accumbens and prefrontal cortex neurons produced by previous experience with amphetamine. *Journal of Neuroscience* 17, 8491-8497.

Rosen, S. (Ed.) (1982) My *Voice Will Go With You: The Teaching Tales of Milton H. Erickson, M.D.* New York, Norton.

Rutter, M. (1982) Syndromes attributed to minimal brain dysfunction in childhood. *American Journal of Psychiatry* 139, 21-33.

Sannerud, C. and Feussner, G. (2000) Is Ritalin an abused drug? Does it meet the criteria of a schedule II substance? In L.L. Greenhill and B.B. Osman (Eds.) *Ritalin: Theory and Practice.* New York: Mary Ann Liebert.

Sax, S. (2000) Living through better chemistry? *The World and I* 15, 287-299.

Schachar, R.J. (1991) Childhood hyperactivity. *Journal of Child Psychology and Psychiatry* 32, 155-191.

Schachar, R., & Tannock, R. (2002). Syndromes of hyperactivity and attention deficit. In M. Rutter and E. Taylor (Eds.) *Child and Adolescent Psychiatry (4th Edition).* Oxford: Blackwell.

Schachter, H., Pham, B., King, J., Langford, S. and Moher, D. (2001) How efficacious and safe is short-acting methylphenidate for the treatment of attention-deficit disorder in children and adolescents? A meta-analysis. *Canadian Medical Association Journal* 165, 1475-1488.

Schmidt, M.H., Esser, G., Allehoff, W., Geisel, B., Laught, M. and Woerner, W. (1987) Evaluating the significance of minimal brain dysfunction - results of an epidemiological study. *Journal of Child Psychology and Psychiatry* 28, 803-821.

Sells, S. (2001) *Parenting your Out of Control Teenager: Seven Steps to Re-establishing Authority and Reclaim Love.* New York: St Martin's Press.

Shazer, S. de (1994) *Words Were Originally Magic.* New York: Norton.

Shen, Y.C., Wong, Y.F. and Yang, X.L. (1985) An epidemiological investigation of minimal brain dysfunction in six elementary schools in Beijing. *Journal of Child Psychology and Psychiatry* 26, 777-788.

Silberg, J., Rutter, M., Meyer, J., et al. (1996) Genetic and environmental influences on the covariation between hyperactivity and conduct disturbance in juvenile twins. *Journal of Child Psychology and Psychiatry* 37, 803-816.

Smith, C. and Nyland, D. (Eds.) (1997) *Narrative Therapies with Children and Adolescents.* New York: The Guildford Press.

Solanto, M.V. and Wender, E.H. (1989) Does Methylphenidate constrict cognitive functioning? *Journal of the American Academy of Child Adolescent Psychiatry* 28, 897-902.

Sonuga-Barke, E.J.S., Minocha, K., Taylor, E.A. and Sandberg, S. (1993) Inter-ethnic bias in teacher's ratings of childhood hyperactivity. *British Journal of Developmental Psychology* 11, 187-200.

Speltz, M.C. (1990) The treatment of preschool conduct problems. In M.T. Greenberg, D. Cicchetti, and E.M. Cummings (Eds.) *Attachment in the Preschool Years.* Chicago: University of Chicago Press.

Spencer, T., Biederman, J., Wilens, T., Harding, M., O'Donnell, D. and Griffin, S. (1996) Pharmacotherapy of attention deficit hyperactivity disorder across the life cycle. *Journal of the American Academy of Child and Adolescent Psychiatry* 35, 409-432.

Sprague, S.L. and Sleator, E.K. (1977) Methylphenidate in hyperkinetic children: Differences in dose effects on learning and social behaviour. *Science* 198, 1274-1276.

Sproson, E.J., Chantrey, J., Hollis, C., Marsden, C.A. and Fonel, K.C. (2001) Effect of repeated methylphenidate administration on presynaptic dopamine and behavior in young adult rats. *Journal of Psychopharmacology* 15, 67-75.

Stein, D.B. (2001) *Unravelling the ADD/ADHD Fiasco: Successful Parenting Without Drugs.* Kansas City: Andrews McMeel.

Stiefle, I. (1997) Can disturbance in attachment contribute to attention deficit hyperactivity disorder? A case discussion. *Clinical Child Psychology and Psychiatry* 2, 45-64.

Still, G.F. (1902) Some abnormal psychiatric conditions in children. *Lancet*, 1008-1012, 1077-1082, 1163-1168.

Strauss, A. and Lehtinen. L. (1947) *Psychopathology and Education of the Brain Injured Child.* New York: Grune and Stratton.

Taylor, E. (1988) Attention deficit and conduct disorder syndromes. In M. Rutter, A.H. Tuma and I.S. Lann (Eds.) *Assessment and Diagnosis in Child Psychopathology.* New York: Guildford Press.

Taylor, E. (1994) Syndromes of attention deficit and over-activity. In M. Rutter, E. Taylor and L. Hersov (Eds.) *Child and Adolescent Psychiatry, Modern Approaches: Third Edition,* Oxford: Blackwell Scientific Publications.

Taylor, E. and Hemsley, R. (1995) Treating hyperkinetic disorders in childhood. *British Medical Journal* 310, 1617-1618.

Taylor, E., Schachar, R., Thorley, G., Weiselberg, H.M., Everitt, B. and Rutter, M. (1987) Which boys respond to stimulant medication? A controlled trial of Methylphenidate in boys with disruptive behaviour. *Psychological Medicine* 17, 121-143.

Thomas, A. and Chess, S. (1977) *Temperament and Development.* New York: Brunner-Mazel.

Timimi, S. (2002) *Pathological Child Psychiatry and the Medicalization of Childhood.* Hove: Brunner-Routledge.

Timimi, S. (2003) The new practitioner. *Young Minds* 62, 14-16.

Timimi, S. (2005) *Naughty Boys: Anti-Social Behaviour, ADHD and the Role of Culture.* Basingstoke: Palgrave MacMillan.

Timimi, S. and 33 co-endorsers (2004) A critique of the international consensus statement on ADHD. *Clinical Child and Family Psychology Review* 7, 59-63.

Tyrer, P. (1996) Co-morbidity or consanguinity. *British Journal of Psychiatry* 168, 669-671.

United States Department of Education (1991) *Memorandum September 16th: Clarification of policy to address the needs of children with Attention Deficit Disorders.* Washington D.C: United States Dept. of Education.

Valenstein, E.S. (1998) *Blaming the Brain.* New York: The Free Press.

Volkow, N.D., Ding, Y.S., Fowler, J.S., et al. (1995) Is Methylphenidate like Cocaine. *Archives of General Psychiatry* 52, 456-463.

Wasserman, R.C., Kelleher, K.J., Bocian, A., et al. (1999) Identification of attentional and hyperactivity problems in primary care: A report from pediatric research in office settings and the ambulatory sentinel practice network. *Pediatrics* 103, E38.

Weis, G., Kruger, E., Danielson, U. and Elman, M. (1975) Effect of long term treatment of hyperactive children with methylphenidate. *Canadian Medical Association Journal* 112, 159-165.

Werry, J.S., Elkind, G.S. and Reeves, J.C. (1987a) Attention deficit, conduct oppositional and anxiety disorders in children. III. Laboratory differences. *Journal of Abnormal Child Psychology* 15, 409-428.

White, M. and Epston, D. (1990) *Narrative Means to Therapeutic Ends.* New York: Norton.

Wolraich, M., Windgren, S., Stromquist, A., Milich, R., Davis, C. and Watson, D. (1990) Stimulant medication use by primary care physicians in the treatment of Attention Deficit Hyperactivity Disorder. *Paediatrics* 86, 95-101.

Wright, O. (2003) Ritalin use and abuse fears. *The Times (UK)* July 28th, 3.

Wurtzel, E. (2002) *More, Now, Again.* London: Virago.

Zahn, T.P., Rapoport, J.L. and Thompson, C.L. (1980) Autonomic and behavioural effects of dextroamphetamine and placebo in normal and hyperactive pre-pubertal boys. *Journal of Abnormal Child Psychology* 8, 145-160.

Zito, J.M., Safer, D.J., Dosreis, S., Gardner, J.F., Boles, J. and Lynch, F. (2000) Trends in prescribing of psychotropic medication in pre-schoolers. *Journal of the American Medical Association* 283, 1025-30.

Zwi, M., Ramchandani, P. and Joughlin, C. (2000) Evidence and belief in ADHD. *British Medical Journal* 321, 975-976.

10
Childhood Depression?

Sami Timimi

Introduction

C hild psychiatry is in desperate need of an interdisciplinary dialogue, the absence of which in the current dominant discourses is leading to faulty assumptions of a bio-deterministic nature and subsequent encouragement of practice that may be worse than useless. At the end of 2003, over 50,000 children were prescribed anti-depressants and over 170,000 prescriptions of anti-depressants per year were being prescribed to under-18s in the UK (Bosely, 2003). The situation in North America is even worse with a sharp rise occurring during the nineties in use of anti-depressants in this age group (Olfson et al, 2002) including the prescribing of antidepressants to pre-school children as young as two (Zito et al, 2000). In December 2003 the UK Committee on Safety in Medicine (CSM), having been forced to re-examine the safety/efficacy profile of the new generation of anti-depressants (the Selective Serotonin Reuptake Inhibitors or SSRIs), issued new guidance to UK doctors stating that these anti-depressants (bar one- fluoxetine) should not be prescribed to the under-18 age group, as available evidence suggests they are not effective and run the risk of serious side effects such as increased suicidality (Ramchandani, 2004). A more recent review (Jureidini et al, 2004) concluded that drug company supported investigators had exaggerated the benefits of the newer anti-depressants in childhood depression and played down adverse effects. They decided that the evidence does not support the use of SSRI anti-depressant drugs (including fluoxetine) for treatment of childhood depression. Older anti-depressants have already been shown not have any beneficial effect in the under 18-age group (Harrington, 1994).

So how did we get into this mess? As Jureidini et al show (2004), part of the problem lays with pharmaceutical industry tactics that are designed to enable greater consumption of their products. The problematic relationship between psychiatry and the drug industry is however more complex than corruption through greed. The gateway diagnosis to prescribing anti-depressants is that of 'childhood depression' a diagnosis that as I show has been borrowed from adult psychiatry and has the effect of cutting the child off from their context. A mutually beneficial relationship between certain academic psychiatrists and the drug industry develops where the psychiatrists give the drug companies the tools and the drug company, by promoting their products, implicitly endorse the validity of the concepts for which their product is being marketed as a 'treatment'. Because anti-depressants are by nature a biological treatment, in order to justify its increasing use, biological explanatory models and research that supports this model, is promoted and childhood depression has thus come to be viewed as a primarily biological problem. A shift in theory and consequently practice took place in the last decade, as influential academics claimed that childhood depression was more common than previously thought (8-20% of children and adolescents), resembled adult depression, and was amenable to treatment with anti-depressants (often resulting in anti-depressants becoming a first line treatment) (Jureidini et al, 2004; Harrington, 1994, Reynolds and Johnston, 1994).

In order to re-examine the concept and usefulness of 'childhood depression', I will address three related questions:

Firstly: Does the concept of 'depression' have cross cultural validity?

Secondly: Is the concept of 'childhood depression' a valid and coherent one?

Thirdly: How useful is the concept of childhood depression when making treatment decisions?

Does the concept of 'depression' have cross-cultural validity?

Reference to anthropological and cross-cultural psychiatric literature throws serious doubt on the cross-cultural validity of the concept of depression as it has been developed and used in Western psychiatry. The concept of depression has been developed with reference to a particular cultural group and when applied to other cultural groups the psychiatric concept of depression lacks coherence and credibility (Kleinman, 1977, 1987; Kleinman and Good, 1985). Many of the key psychiatric symptoms in depression refer to conceptual constructs influenced by Western philosophical ideas. These symptoms may be absent, nonsensical or have entirely different meanings in cultures where different philosophical traditions have been influential, particularly those not governed by notions of a mind/body split (Krause, 1989; Jackson, 1985; Currer, 1986; Obeyesekere, 1985). In order to be able to practice in a non-discriminatory manner in a multi-cultural society, the discrimination inherent in concepts with little cross-cultural validity must be acknowledged and practice must reflect this (Fernando, 1988). Unless we are able to understand the different systems of meaning that exist, we will be faced with a deep-seated problem where the clinician's and the client's paradigms are so incongruent that harmful outcomes can result (Smith, 2003).

The claim is regularly made that the presence of biological markers, such as cortisol hyper-secretion and resistance to the suppressive feedback actions of the synthetic glucocorticoid dexamethasone, in many adults diagnosed with a major depressive disorder, is proof of this condition's primarily biological nature. Whilst such evidence should not be dismissed, it requires a jump in logic to conclude that this is sufficient evidence to confirm the primarily biological underpinnings of depression. Interpreting the meaning of these findings using a more interactive model leads to a more complex appreciation of the interactive nature of the way we acquire subjectivity. For example it is well known that the body secretes more cortisol during times of physical or psychological stress. Thus cortisol hyper-secretion may be better thought of as a marker of physical or environmental stress. Furthermore a complex relationship exists between states of mind and physiological function, which is illustrated by studies that show changes in brain physiology following successful psychological or other environmental interventions. Thus Schwartz et al (1996) demonstrated that when individuals suffering from obsessive compulsive disorder were successfully treated with cognitive behavioural therapy similar changes in brain physiology took place when compared to those successfully treated with an anti-depressant; Rappaport (2003) demonstrated that changes can be seen in the brain physiology of pupils with a diagnosis of dyslexia after undertaking a two week course in remedial reading; and Leuchter et al (2002) has shown that changes can be seen in the brain function of depressed patients successfully treated with a placebo.

This does not negate the importance of a biological perspective, as chronic high cortisol may have an adverse impact on health of body and brain (Goodyer et al, 2001) (as may anti-depressants), but it does require us to abandon simplistic biological reductionism in favour of more interactive models. Interactive approaches also enable us to explore more ecological models that include a biological dimension. Thus depression has been shown to be more prevalent in cultures with a high dietary intake of refined sugar and dairy products and a low intake of fish and seafood (Peet, 2004).

Is the concept of childhood depression a valid and coherent one?

Examining cross-cultural, anthropological, psychological and sociological literature throws up even more question marks over concept of depression in children. Western psychiatry developed within a medical culture with an individualist (as opposed to collectivist) and technological orientation where context (cultural, political, spiritual etc.) has been marginalized (Bracken and Thomas, 2001). Use of such context-depleted paradigms is even more problematic in child psychiatry (Timimi, 2002; 2005) given the dependence children have on adults to make decisions on their behalf (even in the

Western world!). In this section I will discuss how the development of this concept can be viewed as related to two key developments in modernist Western culture, the disappearance of the child/adult boundary and the market economy demand for never ending growth. Following this, I will examine the evidence supporting the suggestion that childhood depression is a biologically based disorder.

Whilst the immaturity of children is a biological fact, the ways in which this immaturity is understood and made meaningful is a fact of culture (Prout and James, 1997). Members of any society carry within themselves a working definition of childhood, its nature, limitations and duration. They may not explicitly discuss this definition, write about it, or even consciously conceive of it as an issue, but they act upon their assumptions in all of their dealings with, fears for, and expectations of their children (Calvert, 1992). Thus our construction of what makes a normal/pathological childhood is not 'innocent' of current political, economic, moral or indeed health concerns. Rather childhood often represents a central arena through which we construct our fantasies about the future and a battleground through which we struggle to express competing ideological agendas.

Before the onset of the Second World War, Western society viewed relations between parents and children primarily in terms of discipline and authority. This pre-war paradigm, grounded in behaviourism, stressed the importance of forming habits of behaviour necessary for productive life. During the Second World War anxiety about the impact on children of discipline and authority began to be expressed, the concern being that 'despotic' discipline could lead to the sort nightmare society that Nazi Germany represented. Scholarly and professional discourses that spoke about the child as an individual and which favoured a more democratic approach to child-rearing, encouraging humane discipline of the child through guidance and understanding, became increasingly popular in political circles and everyday culture (Jenkins, 1998).

The resulting culture of 'permissiveness' represented an ideological response to the Second World War and public distaste for anything smacking of authoritarianism. In addition, whilst the pre-war model prepared children for the workplace within a society of scarcity, the post-war model prepared them to become pleasure-seeking consumers within a prosperous new economy (Wolfenstein, 1955). The post-war 'permissiveness' model saw parent-child relations increasingly in terms of pleasure and play. Parents now had to relinquish traditional authority in order for children to develop autonomy and self-worth.

Childhood, through a process of miniaturization, became a key metaphor through which adults spoke about their social and political concerns. Thus permissiveness with regards child rearing was allowing, not only, new identities to be prescribed for children, but also for adults. Mothers and fathers were responding to this changing definition of childhood and seeing this as a vehicle for fuller expression for themselves. Parental obligations were paving the way for the culture of fun and permissiveness for all.

Shifting economic structures were also leading to profound changes in the organization of family life. More mothers were working and thus a renegotiation of power within the family was taking place. At the same time, suburbanization and the economic demands of successful market economies were resulting in greater mobility, less time for family life and a breakdown of the extended family. Many families (Particularly those headed by young women) were now isolated from traditional sources of childrearing information. In this context childrearing guides took on an unprecedented importance allowing for a more dramatic change in parenting styles than would have been conceivable in a more rooted community, and greater 'ownership' by professionals of the knowledge base for the task of parenting (Zuckerman, 1975). Many parents evaluated their performance according to the new all-but-impossible standards of good childrearing that the parenting manuals written by professionals presented.

The new child-centred permissive culture was a godsend to consumer capitalism. Wall coverings, carpets and furniture were sold to parents on the basis of their child-resistant surfaces. Childhood could now be successfully commercialized and an industry of children's toys, books, and fun educational material developed (Lear, 1963). The culture of consumption (with its expectations of a 'fun morality') became a major force shaping child-rearing practices of the 20th century in the West. With the expansion of the consumer marketplace and suburban affluence, permissive conceptions of the child embraced pleasure as a positive motivation for exploration and learning.

However, critics warned that permissiveness put the parents, especially the mother, at the mercy of the child, who could turn into a 'spoiled brat' and domestic tyrant. In this view of things, the parent in the permissive household became driftwood in the tides of their child's demands. Critics feared we were encouraging small monsters to grow up to become unkempt, irresponsible, destructive, anarchical, drug-oriented and hedonistic non-members of society (Henry, 1963). There was also concern about the changes being wrought on family politics, particularly the role of the father. Thus the fear was that the father could no longer stand for social order in the family and instead was being advised to learn to be playful and have fun with his children. Fathers had to deal with shifting conceptions of gender, male fears of a loss of heroic status, the adoption of greater childrearing responsibilities and a more domestically contained lifestyle. Sadly many fathers started literally taking flight from these new social roles, leading to an enormous growth in single mother families in Western society. Separation and divorce became more common as the permissive discourse of the rights of the individual (to fun and self satisfaction) became stronger than the notion of duties and responsibilities.

Somewhere in the permissive child-centred culture, a hole had opened up in the notion of community and group responsibility and children fell into this. Although a backlash against the culture of permissiveness took place particularly in the 1980's and 90's, it was already too embedded in modern Western notions of childhood. Furthermore this backlash continued to put the individual at the centre and was in service of capital following a period of decline in western economies. More parents were forced to work for longer hours, and state support particularly for children and families was harshly cut resulting in widespread child poverty and the creation of a new under-class.

With the increase in the number of divorces and two working parents, fathers and mothers are around their children for less of the day. A generation of 'home aloners' is growing up; kids who have to by and large raise themselves. As kids are forced to withdraw into their own culture the free market exploits this, praying on their boredom and desire for stimulation (Kincheloe, 1998). In this environment poor children are constantly confronted with their shortcomings by media that tells them they are deficient without this or that accessory. In this unhappy isolation Western children respond to the markets push to 'adultify' them (at the same time as the culture of self-gratification 'childify's' adults) by entering into the world of adult entertainments earlier and without adult supervision. Thus the post-modern Western child is sexually knowledgeable and has early experience of drugs and alcohol (Aronowtiz and Giroux, 1991). Many argue that as a result childhood in the West was being eroded, lost or indeed has suffering a strange death (Jenhs, 1996). It is claimed that childhood is disappearing as children have gained access to the world of adult information resulting in a blurring of boundaries between what is considered adulthood and what is considered childhood, leading to children coming to be viewed as in effect miniature adults.

The result of these competing discourses and changes in family and lifestyle has been the development of some core tensions and ambivalence with regard children. The children's rights movements, see childhood as being at risk and needing safeguarding against pollution by adults (often without noticing how much the permissive, children's rights discourse has already eroded cultural boundaries between adults and children), whilst simultaneously seeing childhood as needing strengthening by developing children's character and ability to reason. In other words, on the one hand childhood needs to be preserved and on the other hand it is made older than its years. This contradiction runs through our modern conception of childhood innocence, we desire it and we want to help children to move beyond it, we want to 'coddle' the child and we want to 'discipline' the child (Aries, 1998).

The growth of the popularity of the concept of childhood depression from a rare to a common diagnosis reflects these broader cultural dynamics. Here we have an individualized notion of little adults falling prey to internal mental diseases that resemble those that effect adults. Children are viewed through a cultural lens that says (and expects) that childhood should be free of any unpleasant emotions. Professionals are viewed as owning the relevant knowledge needed to understand these problems and parents are advised to turn to them for 'objective' appraisal of their children's difficulties.

The political and economic self interest of the medical professional and the pharmaceutical industry has found an ideal set of cultural 'pre-conditions' that can be used to promote context-depleted, biomedical interpretations of childhood problems as well as to bring more experiences previously regarded as ordinary, into the sphere of 'medical problem' (Timimi, 2002; 2005; Double, 2002). Natural and normal human reactions (even if they are undesirable ones) have become too 'dangerous' to allow, particularly if children whom, we are led to believe, should always be protected from anything unpleasant show them. The demands of capital in a market economy means that our culture is gripped by a growth fetish (Hamilton, 2003), whereby new markets have to be developed and more consumption encouraged (Kovel, 2002). It is in this context that new psychiatric diagnoses are continually being invented, numbers of psychiatrists have increased and the amount of psychotropic medication prescribed is rising, seemingly without limit (Double, 2002).

The above should raise concern about the way the concept of childhood depression has evolved, reflecting the tendency to ascribe in a poorly thought out way notions of adult pathology directly onto children. From a purely scientific point of view, it is hard to understand how childhood depression as a diagnosis has come into existence and why it is diagnosed so frequently.

According to the current criteria psychiatric co-morbidity (having more than one diagnosis) in childhood depression is so high, nearly every child can be diagnosed with at least one other psychiatric condition (Harrington, 1994) raising doubts over the specificity of the construct. There is awareness of continuity between 'normal' sadness and 'clinical depression', yet the diagnosis assumes that 'clinical depression' exists as a category (rather than on a continuum) raising questions as to whom and on what basis one decides where the cut-off mark is between 'normal' and 'pathological'. Furthermore, recent studies indicate that having a categorical diagnosis bears only a tenuous relationship with level of psychosocial impairment, with many below a threshold of diagnosis showing higher levels of impairment than those above (Pickles et al, 2001). Similarly childhood depression is only weakly associated with suicide in childhood or adolescence (stronger predictors include history of aggression and use of drugs or alcohol) (Wickes-Nelson and Israel, 2002). The so-called 'biological markers' discussed above that are found in adults do not work with children and adolescents diagnosed as depressed (Harrington, 1994). With regards genetics, separating environmental from biological factors in the familial clustering has been virtually impossible, particularly as the offspring of parents diagnosed with depression are at risk of developing a wide range of psychiatric disorders (Wickes-Nelson and Israel, 2002).

Much has been made about the suggested continuity of childhood depression into adulthood and thus it has been argued that childhood depression is a precursor of adulthood depression (Harrington, 1990). The emerging picture is more confusing. Firstly, only a small number who meet the criteria for childhood depression are diagnosed with depression as adults (Kolvin et al, 1991). Secondly, follow-up studies have used dubious standards for diagnosing adult psychiatric disorders (for example symptoms that need to be present for 4 weeks only), have discovered high rates of co-morbidity (when they were children and again as adults), have been unable to differentiate biological factors from continuing social adversity (Harrington et al, 1993; Fombonne et al, 2001) and have not taken into account the possible effects of any treatment received (in other words the possibility that continuing morbidity may be due to the toxic side effects of medications taken and/or effect on self-worth together with the psychosocial adversity that arises as a result of becoming a 'psychiatric patient').

So despite little evidence to support the existence of a discrete, naturally occurring, entity called 'childhood depression', it slipped into psychiatric and then every day medical nosology as if it were an already proven fact. Following on from my suggestion that one social dynamic behind the rise in the popularity of this construct is the 'adultifying' of childhood, leading researchers began to claim that childhood depression resembles adult depression (Harrington, 1994). However, based on symptoms alone it is clear that children do not show many of the symptoms said to be common in adult depression (such as loss of weight and appetite, sleep disturbance and feelings of guilt). Instead more non-specific symptoms such as irritability, running away from home, decline in schoolwork and headaches are described as indicative of childhood depression (Hill, 1997).

In conclusion then, the birth and increasing popularity of the diagnosis of childhood depression reflects the effects of a wider socio-cultural process occurring in Western society (of a diminishing boundary between the way we conceive childhood and adulthood, together with the economic need to create and expand new markets), rather than being the result of any medical breakthrough.

How useful is the concept of childhood depression when it comes to making treatment decisions?

The problem with context-deprived notions of childhood problems (such as childhood depression) is that they lead to context-deprived, often medicalized, solutions of dubious value and that may carry considerable risks. This has resulted in a dramatic increase in the inappropriate use of anti-depressants in children and adolescents.

The current state of evidence with regards the efficacy of anti-depressants in children and adolescents is clear. There is no convincing evidence that anti-depressants show any benefit over placebo in children or adolescents (Ambrosini et al, 1993; Hazell et al, 1995; 2002). Studies that claim to have demonstrated a small benefit over placebo were on clinician measures only, patient and carer measures did not demonstrate any improved outcome over placebo (Emslie et al, 1997; Avci et al, 1999 and see chapter 2). When we couple this evidence (or lack of it) with the deep concerns that exist about potentially fatal side effects (whether through cardio-toxicity or provoking suicidal impulses) and our lack of knowledge concerning the possible effects antidepressants have on the developing brain, the implications are clear.

It should be noted that there remains considerable doubt with regards the efficacy of anti-depressants in adults. There is considerable evidence to suggest that in adults anti-depressant drug effects are not much greater than placebo, particularly when compared to an active placebo (Greenberg and Fisher, 1997; Healy, 1999; Moncrieff, 2002), that psychological treatments are at least as effective as pharmacotherapy, even in severe depression and especially if patient rated and long term measures are used (Antonuuccio et al, 1995, 1997; De Rubeis et al, 1999), and that pharmacotherapy alone increases vulnerability to relapse (Hollon et al, 1991; Segal et al, 1999).

The increase in rates of childhood depression in Western culture (Rutter and Smith, 1995; Fombonne, 1995) in recent years may well reflect a lowering of the threshold for the diagnosis due to the medicalization of childhood problems. However, part of the reason may also be a genuine increase in unhappiness being experienced by children having to grow up in a cultural context that has seen huge changes in child rearing practices, family structure, lifestyle, and education. In the latter half of the last century there was a marked increase in the rates of psychosocial problems (such as crime, suicidal behaviour, anxiety, depression, and substance abuse) amongst children and adolescents in Western societies (Rutter and Smith, 1995). Much evidence exists to suggest that children and adolescents in the West experience greater mental health problems as a result of the adverse impact on them of socio-cultural changes. For example, an increase in family decay (from factors such as divorce rates) is associated with increases in youth violence, substance abuse and suicide (Pampei, 2001).

What a context-deprived approach allows our profession to collude with, are the de-politicisation of children's difficulties and the obscuring of the changing challenges facing children and their families in modern Western capitalist societies. In a culture characterized by a growth fetish, where adults are channelled into the endless pursuit of individualistic self-gratification, children get in the way. The increase in rates of 'childhood depression' in Western culture in recent years may well reflect increasing unhappiness being experienced by children having to grow up in a cultural context that does not value them.

Their real life circumstances (including biological factors such as diet, exercise and cognitive abilities) need integrating into a multi-perspective approach that engages with the interpersonal realities experienced and the new possible meanings that can be generated when the reliance on reductionistic models that emphasise pathology are abandoned in favour of more positive approaches (such as building on existing strengths and resilience). Indeed in my clinical practice as a full time consultant child and adolescent psychiatrist in the UK, it has been a long time (years) since I last needed to use an anti-depressant.

Conclusion

The escalating use of antidepressants in children and adolescents, despite the absence of any evidence with regards their efficacy in this age group and the major concerns that exist with regards their dangerous side-effects, should make us pause to consider how such an apparently unhelpful medical response to children's unhappiness came about. I argue that the central problem lies in the development of a medicalized notion of 'childhood depression', which can be understood as being the result of cultural dynamics such as the disappearing boundary between notions of childhood and adulthood and the market economy imperative of unlimited growth. Deprived of readily available extended family, parents have increasingly turned to professionals for guidance on child rearing, who in turn have taken ownership of the 'common' knowledge on how to rear children. From here psychiatrists have taken ownership of children's unhappiness, turned this into a medical disorder with an assumption that this disorder has a biological origin, thus providing drug companies with the ideal tools they needed to open up mass markets in the prescription of antidepressants (mainly via general practitioners) to under-18s.

Medical researchers need to develop a more creative dialogue with researchers from other disciplines (such as sociology) to integrate within-body perspectives with broader ones. Childhood depression as an individualised, context-depleted label that offers little explanatory power and can marginalise more helpful, context-rich explanations; may first need to be abandoned before more comprehensive theory and practice with regards to children's unhappiness can emerge.

References

Ambrosini P.J., Bianchi M.D., Rabinovich H., Elia J. (1993) Antidepressant treatments in children and adolescents. I. Affective disorders. *Journal of the American Academy of Child and Adolescent Psychiatry* 32, 1-6.

Antonuccio D.O., Danton W.G., DeNelsky G.Y. (1995) Psychotherapy versus medication for depression: challenging the conventional wisdom with data. Professional *Psychology: Research and Practice* 26, 574-585.

Antonuccio D.O., Thomas M., Danton W.G. (1997) A cost-effectiveness analysis of cognitive behavior therapy and fluoxetine (Prozac) in the treatment of depression. *Behavior Therapy* 28, 187-210.

Aries P. (1998) From immodesty to innocence. In H Jenkins (ed.), *Children's Culture Reader*. New York: New York University Press.

Aronowitz S., Giroux H. (1991) *Post-modern Education: Politics, Culture and Social Criticism*. Minneapolis: University of Minnesota Press.

Avci A., Diler R.S., Kibar M., Sezgin F. (1999), Comparison of moclobemide and placebo in young adolescents with major depressive disorder. *Annals of Medical Science* 8, 31-40.

Boseley S. (2003) 50,000 children taking antidepressants. *The Guardian* 20th September.

Bracken P., Thomas P. (2001) Post psychiatry: a new direction for mental health. *British Medical Journal* 322, 724-727.

Calvert, K. (1992) *Children in the House: The Material Culture of Early Childhood, 1600-1900*. Boston: Northeastern University Press.

Currer C. (1986) Concepts of mental and ill being: The case of Pathan mothers in Britain. In C. Currer, M. Stacey (eds.) *Concepts of Health, Illness and Disease: A Comparative Perspective*. Lemington Spa: Berg.

DeRubeis R.J., Gelfand L.A., Tang T.Z., Simons A.D. (1999) Medications versus cognitive behavior therapy for severely depressed outpatients: mega-analysis of four randomized comparisons. *American Journal of Psychiatry* 156, 1007-1013.

Double D. (2002) The limits of psychiatry. *British Medical Journal* 324, 900-904.

Emslie G.J., Rush A.J., Weinberg W.A. et al. (1997) A double-blind, randomized, placebo-controlled trial of fluoxetine in children and adolescents with depression. *Archives of General Psychiatry* 54, 1031-1037.

Fernando S. (1988) *Race and Culture in Psychiatry*. London: Croom Helm.

Fombonne E. (1995) Depressive disorders: time trends and possible explanatory mechanisms. In M. Rutter, D.J. Smith (eds.) *Psychosocial Disorders in Young People: Time Trends and their Causes*. Chichester: John Wiley and Sons.

Fombonne E., Wostear G., Cooper V., Harrington R., Rutter M. (2001) The Maudsley long-term follow-up of child and adolescent depression 1. Psychiatric outcomes in adulthood. *British Journal of Psychiatry* 179, 210-217.

Goodyer I.M., Park R.J., Netherton C., Herbert J. (2001) Possible role of cortisol and dehydroepiandrosterone in human development and psychopathology. *British Journal of Psychiatry* 179, 243-249.

Greenberg R.P., Fisher S. (1997) Mood-mending medicines: probing drug, psychotherapy, and placebo solutions. In S Fisher, RP Greenberg (eds.) *From Placebo to Panacea: Putting Psychiatric Drugs to the Test*. New York: John Wiley.

Hamilton C. (2003) *Growth Fetish*. Crows Nest: Allen and Unwin.

Harrington R. (1994) Affective disorders. In M. Rutter, E. Taylor, L. Hersov (eds.) *Child and Adolescent Psychiatry, Modern Approaches: Third Edition*. Oxford: Blackwell Scientific Publications.

Harrington R., Fudge H., Rutter M., Bredenkamp C., Groothues C., Pridham J. (1993) Child and adult depression: A test of continuities with data from a family study. *British Journal of Psychiatry* 162, 627-633.

Hazell P., O'Connell D., Heathcote D. (1995) Efficacy of tricyclic drugs in treating child and adolescent depression: a meta-analysis. *British Medical Journal* 310, 897-901.

Hazell P., O'Connell D., Heathcote D., Henry D. (2002) Tricyclic drugs for depression in children and adolescents. *Cochrane Database Systematic Revue* CD002317.

Healy D. (1999) *The Antidepressant Era*. Cambridge, MA: Harvard University Press.

Henry J. (1963) *Culture Against Man*. New York: Vintage.

Hill P. (1997) Child and adolescent psychiatry. In R. Murray, P. Hill, P. McGuffin (eds.) *The Essentials of Postgraduate Psychiatry: Third Edition*. Cambridge: Cambridge University Press.

Hollon S.D., Shelton R.C., Loosen P.T. (1991) Cognitive therapy and pharmacotherapy for depression. *Journal of Consultative Clinical Psychology* 59, 88-99.

Jackson S. (1985) Acedia, the sins and its relationship to sorrow and melancholia. In A. Kleinman, B. Good (eds.) *Culture and Depression*. Berkley: University of California Press.

Jenhs C. (1996) *Childhood*. London: Routledge.

Jenkins, H. (1998) Introduction: Childhood innocence and other modern myths. In H. Jenkins (ed.) *Children's Culture Reader*. New York: New York University Press.

Jureidini J., Doecke C., Mansfield P.R., Haby M., Menkes D.B., Tonkin A. (2004) Efficacy and safety of antidepressants for children and adolescents. *British Medical Journal* 328, 879-883.

Kincheloe J. (1998) The new childhood; Home alone as a way of life. In H. Jenkins (ed.) *Children's Culture Reader*. New York: New York University Press.

Kleinman A. (1977) Depression, somatization and the new cross-cultural psychiatry. *Social Science and Medicine* 11, 3-10.

Kleinman A. (1987) Anthropology and Psychiatry. The role of culture in cross cultural research on illness. *British Journal of Psychiatry* 151, 447-454.

Kleinman A., Good B. (1985) Introduction: Culture and depression. In A Kleinman, B Good (eds.) *Culture and Depression*. Berkley: University of California Press.

Kolvin I., Barret M.L., Bhate S.R., Berney T.P., Famuyiwa O., Fundudis T., Tyrer S. (1991) The Newcastle child depression project: diagnosis and classification of depression. *British Journal of Psychiatry* 159 (Supplement 11), 9-21.

Kovel J. (2002) *The Enemy of Nature: The End of Capitalism or the End of the World?* London: Zed Books.

Krause I. (1989) Sinking heart: A Punjabi communication of distress. *Social Science and Medicine* 29, 563-575.

Lear M.W. (1963) *The Child Worshipers.* New York: Pocket.

Leuchter A.F., Cook L.A., Witte E.A. (2002) Changes in brain function of depressed patients during treatment with placebo. *American Journal of Psychiatry* 159, 122-129.

Moncrieff J. (2002) The antidepressant debate. *British Journal of Psychiatry* 180, 193-194

Obeyesekere G. (1985) Depression, Buddhism and the work of culture in Sri Lanka. In A. Kleinman, B. Good (eds.) *Culture and Depression.* Berkley: University of California Press.

Olfson M., Marcus S.C., Weissman M.M., Jensen P.S. (2002) National trends in the use of psychotropic medications by children. *Journal of the American Academy of Child and Adolescent Psychiatry* 41, 514-21.

Pampei F., (2001) Williamson J. Age Patterns of Suicide and Homicide Mortality Rates in High-Income Nations. *Social Forces* 80, 251-282.

Peet M. (2004) International variations in the outcome of schizophrenia and the prevalence of depression in relation to national dietary practices: an ecological analysis. *British Journal of Psychiatry* 184, 404-408.

Pickles A., Rowe R., Simonoff E., Foley D., Rutter M., Silberg J. (2001) Child psychiatric symptoms and psychosocial impairment: relationship and prognostic significance. *British Journal of Psychiatry* 179, 230-253.

Prout A., James A. (1997) A new Paradigm for the sociology of childhood? Provenance, promise and problems. In A. James, A. Prout (eds.) *Constructing and Re-constructing Childhood: Contemporary Issues in the Sociological Study of Childhood.* London: Falmer Press.

Ramchandani P. (2004) Treatment of major depressive disorder in children and adolescents. *British Medical Journal* 328, 3-4.

Rappaport J. (2003) Cornell improves the brain. Stratiawire.com February, 2003.

Rutter M., Smith D. (1995) *Psychosocial Disorders in the Young: Time Trends and their causes.* Chichester: John Wiley and Sons.

Reynolds W.M., Johnston H.F. (1994) *Handbook of Depression in Children and Adolescents.* New York: Plenum Press.

Schwartz J.M., Stoessel P.W., Baxter L.R., Karron M. (1996) Systematic changes in cerebral glucose metabolic rate after successful behaviour modification treatment of obsessive-compulsive disorder. *Archives of General Psychiatry* 53, 109-113.

Segal Z.V., Gemar M., Williams S. (1999) Differential cognitive response to a mood challenge following successful cognitive therapy or pharmacotherapy for unipolar depression. *Journal of Abnormal Psychology* 108, 3-10.

Smith R. (2003) An extreme failure of concordance. *British Medical Journal* 327, 818.

Timimi S. (2002) *Pathological Child Psychiatry and the Medicalization of Childhood.* London: Brunner-Routledge.

Timimi S. (2005) *Naughty Boys: Anti-Social Behaviour, ADHD, and the Role of Culture.* Basingstoke: Palgrave MacMillan.

Wickes-Nelson R., Israel A. (2002) *Behaviour Disorders of Childhood.* London: Pearson Higher Education.

Wolfenstein M. (1955) Fun morality: An analysis of recent child-training literature. In M. Mead, M. Wolfenstein (eds.) *Childhood in Contemporary Cultures.* Chicago: The University of Chicago Press.

Zito J.M., Safer D.J., Dosreis S., Gardner J.F., Boles J., Lynch F. (2000) Trends in prescribing of psychotropic medication in pre-schoolers. *Journal of the American Medical Association* 283, 1025-30.

Zuckerman M. (1975) Dr. Spock: The Confidence Man. In S. Kaplan, C. Rosenberg (eds) *The Family in History.* Philadelphia: University of Pennsylvania Press.

11
The Cactus Clinic – An integrative approach to the treatment of ADHD

David Woodhouse

Introduction

The Cactus Clinic was founded in 2000 by the late Professor Steven Baldwin and operated for a year before his untimely death in the Selby rail disaster. The Clinic re-opened in February 2003 and continues to function with the underlying philosophy of offering a non-medication approach to the treatment of ADHD.

The Clinic serves as an information, treatment and research centre. The need for information became apparent at a number of levels. Many parents who came to the Clinic had been told that, unless they placed their child on medication, there was nothing else that the medical profession could do for them, as this was the only treatment on offer for ADHD. Other parents had been told that if they wanted their child to remain in school then they must put him on a medication programme, and those who had followed the medical advice were given little or no information about the potential side effects of the medication. Similarly, parents with children on the medication programme had seen these side effects and wanted to take their child off medication. For these parents a common cry was 'I want my child back' while he is on medication 'there is nobody there!' Parents come to the Clinic seeking an alternative approach to the management of their child's behaviour.

It is evident that for the past 40 years the majority of the medical establishment has ignored the possible link between nutrition and physical disease states. Similarly, the mental health community has followed their lead, with mainstream psychiatry and psychology maintaining there is little relationship between nutrition and supposed mental conditions. Yet a review of the literature reveals that, for virtually every major mental condition, studies exist demonstrating that there are significant nutritional influences (Holford, 2003). It appears that there is a kind of schizophrenia on the part of many mental health practitioners, with their perceptions at odds with research evidence.

The unfortunate reality is that just because there are important discoveries, with the results being replicated many times, there is no guarantee that any changes will take place. Where new findings conflict with traditional beliefs, it is generally the situation that the beliefs continue to dominate for a considerable time. In reality, it is often the belief in an approach, rather than its validity and efficacy that makes for its continued use. Consequently, there is the phenomenon of traditional approaches dying an extended death; these outdated treatments are frequently terminal but never seem to completely expire. They seem to be supported by, at best, a lack of awareness by some members of the medical profession or, at worst, medical megalomania and conceit.

This appears to be the case concerning the issues involved in the debate surrounding the diagnosis and management of ADHD. A fundamental concern is that an ADHD 'diagnosis' is a descriptive label for a particular collection of behavioural and learning difficulties with no indication as to possible causes. No evidence has been found to support the idea that ADHD represents any definite 'disease' with a single biological cause (NIH Consensus Statement, 1998). The issue of co morbidity is central given the number of behavioural and learning difficulties that this diagnosis covers can differ considerably between individuals. Research evidence suggests that 50%-80% of children with a diagnosis of ADHD meets the criteria for a least one other different diagnosis (Biederman, 2004).

There are many physical medical conditions that have similar symptoms as ADHD, and they are not always considered before a diagnosis is made. These include some genetic conditions, hormonal and metabolic disorders, infectious diseases or neurological disorders as well as metal intoxications or serious nutritional deficiencies.

An ADHD diagnosis cannot be considered in isolation. A wide range of other psychiatric conditions needs to be taken into account, such as depression or bipolar disorder, anxiety disorders, obsessive-compulsive disorder and Tourette's syndrome. Other psychiatric diagnoses that may apply include 'oppositional defiant disorder' or 'conduct disorder', and there can be considerable overlap with ADHD. Unfortunately they are subject to a similar debate questioning whether they are 'medical' conditions, with a true physical basis, as these kinds of behavioural problems usually reflect a complex array of social, cultural, economic and other influences (Baldwin, 2000a). Similarly, individuals diagnosed with ADHD often have co morbid learning difficulties such as dyslexia and dyspraxia. This overlap can be as high as 50%, and although each of these conditions can occur individually this is often not the case (Rasmussen and Gillberg, 2000).

This concept of co morbidity is an essential feature in the treatment of ADHD. Children with different co morbidity patterns respond differently to specific treatments and often demonstrate unique outcomes. (Achenbach, 1991) There is ample evidence to suggest that most treatments believed by the medical profession to be effective for ADHD (predominantly stimulants) do not significantly improve depression. There is evidence to suggest that there is a possibility that stimulant medication may increase the number of negative side effects (DuPaul et al., 1994). In addition, treatments for mood disorders are generally not helpful for ADHD. Furthermore, in the presence of a co morbid mood disorder, the stimulants themselves are less effective for ADHD. No stimulant treatments that are noradrenergic but not serotonergic are effective for ADHD. In contrast, serotonergic antidepressants are felt to be effective for juvenile depression but not for ADHD. When considered specifically for ADHD, stimulants are thought to be ineffective on behaviour for more than 25% of children and this can rise to 70% in a co morbid condition with anxiety. (Buitelaar et al., 1995)

It is interesting to note that research into the area of the neurotransmitter systems in the brain have recognized how these are involved in mental health and this has been reflected in subsequent treatment by the medical profession. Although a substantial number of neurotransmitters have been identified there are four main ones that have been the most carefully studied and are thought to be associated with the majority of mental health problems – Dopamine, Serotonin, Norepinephrine, and GABA (Gamma Aminobutyric Acid). Too much or too little of these neurotransmitters is felt to be related to a number of conditions such as depression, bi-polar disorder, ADHD, and schizophrenia. Indeed, most of the drugs used in the treatment of these conditions are reputed to work on these neurotransmitters. For example, methylphenidate (marketed as Ritalin or Concerta) is the leading medication associated with ADHD. Its mode of action is thought to be linked to the dopamine neurotransmitter system. Psychiatric conditions such as paranoia and schizophrenia are treated with medications that are believed to block or lower dopamine in the brain.

Similarly, atomoxetine, now marketed as Strattera and seen as an alternative medication for ADHD, is reported to work on the norepinephrine neurotransmitter system. Most of the medications used for the treatment of depression are thought to be linked to the serotonin neurotransmitter system as are the medications used for the treatment of bulimia, anorexia, social anxiety and phobias in general. GABA is a neurotransmitter that acts as an inhibitor, that is, it affects the ability of the other neurotransmitters to function effectively. Low levels of GABA are associated with problems of poor impulse control and associated with epilepsy and seizure disorders. Thus medications for seizures, impulse control problems and bi-polar disorder all work by increasing the GABA levels. Such drugs as lithium and anti-seizure medications all increase GABA. The medical profession has no difficulty in accepting the above ideas in terms of the impact that the neurotransmitter systems have on psychiatric conditions.

A more detailed examination of the neurotransmitter system from a nutritional perspective is interesting. The basic ingredients for the neurotransmitter system are amino acids that are taken into the body through food. There are eight essential amino acids from which all other amino acids can be made which the brain and body need to function effectively. Neurotransmitters are made from amino acids derived from these eight. For example, dopamine is made from tyrosine, as are norepinephrine and epinephrine. Serotonin is made from the amino acid tryptophan whereas GABA is derived from taurasine. Having the right balance of these neurotransmitters is essential for mental health. But having the right balance of these is not enough in that there are 45 essential nutrients; 20 are minerals, 15 vitamins, and two essential fats in addition to the eight amino acids. The body cannot make these so they must be obtained from food. Not only must they be obtained from food but also they are all interdependent, they all work in synergy (Holford, 1997). Some nutrients will not be effective without their partner substance(s).

Essential Fatty Acids (EFAs) are fundamental to existence, without them the body will slowly degenerate and ultimately die. They are needed for the transport and turning of food into energy for all the body's activities. They are needed for brain development and functioning (Crawford, 2000); they are also needed in the cells and the structures surrounding the cells (Nunez, 1993). But if EFAs are to have the required outcomes, they must work with a number of nutrient partners. Magnesium, biotin, iron, zinc, ascorbic acid and vitamins B3, B6 and C must be present in adequate amounts for normal functioning of EFAs. Similarly, the vitamin B6 is virtually useless until a zinc-dependent enzyme converts it. So an individual who is zinc deficient and taking a B6 supplement for a particular problem will not experience any beneficial effects (Arnold et al., 2000).

In the same way, minerals work together and work with other nutrients to maintain a healthy individual. Calcium, which is essential for bone growth, heart muscle function and the substance holding body cells together, requires magnesium, which helps transmit nerve impulses to muscles, for absorption and use. Iron, which is essential for the oxygen-carrying constituent of blood, needs copper to ensure its efficient absorption from food.

Nutrients are therefore very sensitive to the conditions and contributions under which they are consumed. Further research has indicated that these nutrients may also have a significant impact on behaviour. Studies indicate a mix of positive changes to the child that result from manipulations of diet and nutrition. Broadly, the areas in which significant improvement was witnessed were in behaviour, attention (visual and auditory) and mood. Harding, Judah and Grant (2003) found a significant increase in ratings of visual and auditory performance amongst children administered a dietary supplement (containing vitamins, phytonutrients, amino acids, essential fatty acids, phospholipids and probiotics) equal to that of the improvement seen in children administered Ritalin prior to testing. Peisser and Buitelaar (2002) witnessed improvements in behaviours as rated on the Connors ADHD rating scale following an elimination diet. Improvements in mood are also seen in children with ADHD following nutritional changes, especially in overall irritability, restlessness and inattention (Dengate, 2002).

There is mounting evidence that children with behavioural problems are sensitive to one or more food components that can negatively impact on their behaviour (Schnoll, 2003). This hypersensitivity may be a cause or a symptom of ADHD, or it may be one factor in a rich network of psychological and social factors that accumulates to an attention problem. Dommisse (2000), Cushman (2001) and Ghiora (2003) all highlight the role of nutrition in attention with Ghiora going on to express grave misgivings about the level of information given to parents regarding nutritional information and the link between nutrition and ADHD.

A study by Burgess (2000) linked the behavioural improvements associated with nutritional changes to Long-Chain Polyunsaturated Fatty Acids (LCP). He stated that the symptoms of ADHD were also present in people with essential fatty acid (EFA) deficiencies. The suggestion that ADHD is somehow linked to a deficit in fatty acids is a common theme. Stordy (2000) supports the findings of Burgess; suggesting children with ADHD are missing LCP; Kidd (2003) also found that a nutritional supplement containing amongst other things 6 essential fatty acids, omega-3 and omega-4 would ameliorate the symptoms of ADHD as did Stevens (2003). Ross (2003) reported significant high levels of ethane (a measure of oxidative damage of n-3 fatty acids), which he argued reflects higher than average rates of oxidative breakdown of n-3 polyunsaturated fatty acids in children with ADHD. The work of Richardson (2002) fully endorses the role of essential fatty acids in a number of conditions.

In light of the increasing debate over the diagnosis and management of ADHD, the Clinic offers three programmes; a drug withdrawal programme, a nutritional assessment and guidance programme and the Caregivers skills programme.

The Drug withdrawal programme

The drug withdrawal programme provides a safe withdrawal process from prescribed drugs. For children and teenagers who have been prescribed medication as a treatment for ADHD, all medication is withdrawn. This process is straightforward, but not quick. It takes usually two to four months depending on the dosage and as many children being medicated for ADHD and related problems are on a cocktail of psychiatric drugs, each child is treated as an individual.

The Nutritional Programme

The Nutritional protocol of The Cactus Clinic aims to identify and correct biochemical imbalances. An initial in depth nutritional consultation with the family investigates holistic health to include past medical history, incorporating any pre-conceptual or developmental influences, current health problems, medication, diet and lifestyle.

Food intolerances are identified using a simple pinprick of the finger. The laboratory screens for IgG[1] antibodies in the blood against a panel of 76 foods. Once identified the foods are removed from the diet for a minimum of three months. This allows the antibodies to die and the digestive wall to heal. It is the deficiencies in the EFA that cause the 'leaky' gut. When undigested food goes through a leaky gut into the blood stream the immune system sees it as a threat and attacks. This is the cause of allergic reactions.

Many of the children treated in the Clinic for ADHD type symptoms have a history of repeated ear and upper respiratory infections in early life leading to frequent antibiotic therapy. Antibiotics destroy the friendly gut flora causing a dysbiosis (imbalance) of gut flora and a porous gut wall. This assault on the wall of the digestive tract may then allow food proteins to enter the blood stream and initiate food intolerances (Holman, 1998).

Tissue minerals are determined using an analysis of hair; while this is contentious in orthodox medicine, it is used in forensic medicine with credibility. New hair growth is a better indicator of tissue mineral levels than blood levels. Children with behaviours classified as ADHD appear to have low levels of calcium, magnesium, zinc and manganese: all crucial for optimum nerve transmission. In addition, heavy metal toxicity is identified, elevated levels of mercury, cadmium and aluminium are also commonly found. Correction of deficiencies or excesses can be achieved with supplementation of minerals and vitamins.

The presence of krytopyrroles in urine identifies a condition known as Pyroluria. An abnormal production of a group of chemicals called pyrroles increases the need for zinc and B6. Pyrolurics often have insomnia, hyperactivity, poor memory, poor cognitive function, depression and fatigue.

The nutritional strategy implemented by the Cactus Clinic includes a five-step approach:

1 Balancing blood sugar levels
2 Eliminating chemical additives, preservatives and other allergens
3 Supplementation of fatty acids
4 Correcting nutritional deficiencies of minerals and vitamins
5 Test for and eliminate toxic elements

---

[1] IgG: Food intolerance symptoms are thought to be reactions involving immunoglobin G (IgG). These food intolerance symptoms rarely occur immediately but can be delayed over a period of time and so are difficult to detect. This test measures the levels of food specific IgG of an individual as a means of differentiating an intolerance from an allergic reaction where the latter usually occurs very quickly with an obvious reaction.

The balancing of blood sugar levels is essential and managed by removing refined carbohydrates and stimulants, such as sugar and caffeine. A plant based diet rich in whole foods and complex carbohydrates is balanced with protein, half as much protein as carbohydrate with every food and snack. Additionally, eating a breakfast and never going for more than three hours without food may maintain blood sugar levels within normal parameters. Adequate levels of chromium and B vitamins are required for glucose tolerance.

The programme automatically advocates removing all chemical additives, preservatives and bulking agents. This involves working with parents and providing literature regarding these additives. Those foods for which the individual has tested positive are removed from the diet for a period of time ranging from three months to one year.

The supplementation of EFAs is considered as essential (Richardson, 2003) and Omega 3 and Omega 6 are the main supplements used on a regular basis. The supplementation is augmented with an adequate supply of the key nutrients that have been discussed is essential. Although the changes in diet will ultimately make up for deficiencies initially a number of additional nutrients may be required based on each individual's tests results.

The fifth stage involves the elimination of toxic elements, including heavy metals and parasites, and correcting gut dysbiosis is necessary. Repairing gut permeability with glutamine, liver support and detoxification may also be required.

The advantage of this nutritional approach to the management of ADHD is the recognition of co morbidity and the synergy of the nutritional system. As previously stated, ADHD has many overlapping conditions ranging from various mood disorders to learning difficulties. Unfortunately there appears to be very little overlap in the diagnosis and management of these conditions by the medical professions.

Sam – A case study

Sam is an example of the child that has attended the Clinic. He came to the Clinic aged 11 and weighing five stones. He had been a difficult birth and was on formula milk after three days and had had mild eczema as a child. He had been diagnosed with ADHD at the age of seven after exhibiting problem behaviour for a number of years. He had problems with aggressive behaviour in school and his academic work suffered. His mother coped well with him at home. She had resisted the efforts of both the school and the psychiatrist to have put him on medication and had tried a number of alternative approaches including hypnotherapy and anger management. Finally, under the threat of exclusion from school he was put on Ritalin at the age of nine. His medication was only given on schooldays and never at weekends or holidays. Whilst on medication he did not eat well and developed nervous tics and appeared 'spaced out'. His school said he worked really well when he was on Ritalin. Concerned about the side effects his parents slowly withdrew him from Ritalin and by the time he started at the Clinic he was down to 5mg per day. His initial TOVA[2] scores indicated that he did have problems with attention and impulsivity. The charts below give a pictorial representation of his performance when he was first tested in the Clinic. His scored 135 on the TOVA behavioural checklist at the beginning of the programme.

A full nutritional assessment was undertaken. The food intolerance test results showed that Sam had milk, wheat and gluten intolerances. His nutrient mineral check showed that he had low magnesium, calcium and copper levels with excessively high iron and chromium levels. Mineral balance is as important as the mineral levels and Sam's mineral imbalance test indicated that he had significantly high zinc/copper, sodium/magnesium, calcium/magnesium and copper/iron ratios. Conversely he had significantly low sodium/potassium and sodium/calcium ratio levels. Sam also demonstrated high levels of arsenic and aluminium.

The overall aim of the nutritional programme was to restore the mineral levels and mineral balances to their optimum levels and remove the foods to which he had intolerance. The programme followed the five-point plan outlined earlier. He was also given a course of nutritional supplements to counter the imbalances both in the diet and the mineral content.

Sam was retested on the TOVA three months later. His scores were no longer in the ADHD range and a comparison of the pre and post-test charts give some indication of the change that had taken place in the three-month period. His score on the TOVA behaviour checklist had dropped to 91.

Comparison of Sam's Pre and Post Test Scores on the TOVA

The following charts give some idea of the changes that Sam has made in a three-month period in terms of both his attention and impulsive behaviour. High scores indicate a positive change. The bars represent scores achieved on the four quarters of the test, followed by the scores for the two halves of the test and then the total score.

---

[2] TOVA is a continuous performance test entitled Test of Variables of Attention developed by Lawrence Greenberg. It is used as a tool in the clinic to assess a child's attention levels and impulsivity. Although it gives a score for ADHD it is not used as a diagnostic test but as one of the ways of determining the effectiveness of the programmes.

PRE – TEST	POST – TEST

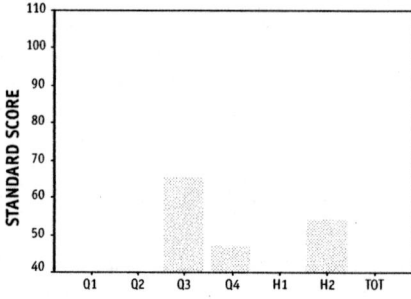

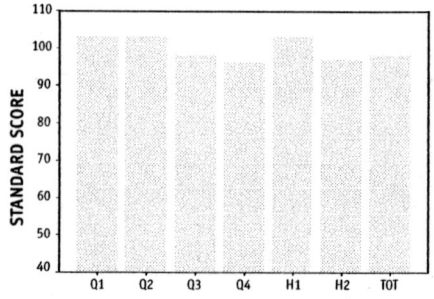

OMISSION (INATTENTION)   OMISSION (INATTENTION)

Errors in omission can be viewed as a measure of attention and happen when the child does not press the button when the target appears. In Sam's case, on the pre-test, it is clear that his omissions were extensive and his attention 'window' could be considered negligible. Three months later there is a marked improvement with a 'normal' window of attention.

PRE – TEST	POST – TEST

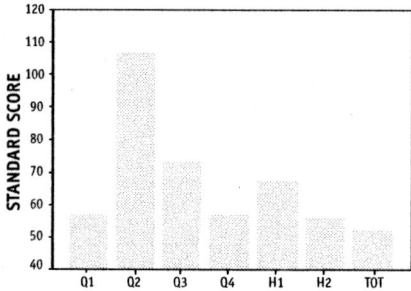

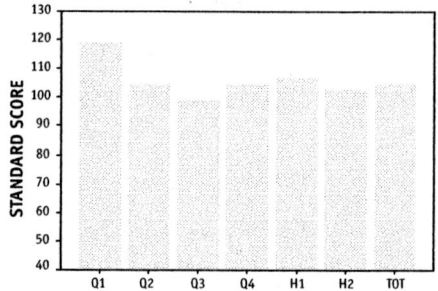

COMMISSION (IMPULSIVITY)   COMMISSION (IMPULSIVITY)

Commission errors are considered to be a measure of impulsivity and occur when the child pushes the button when they should not do so. In Sam's pre-test it is clear that he some problems with impulsivity with the low number of correct responses. Again there is a marked improvement in the post test.

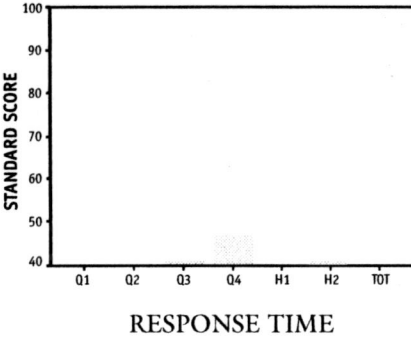

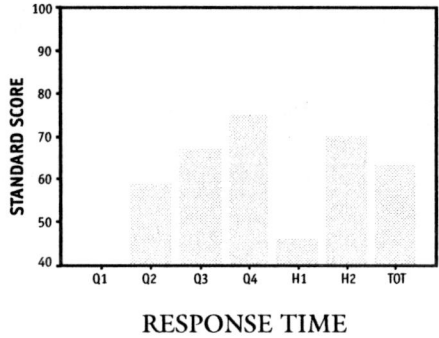

RESPONSE TIME   RESPONSE TIME

The response time is the processing speed that it takes to respond correctly to the target. Children with ADD often have slower than normal response times rather than faster ones. Once again it can be seen that there has been a significant improvement in Sam's scores although there is still room for more improvement.

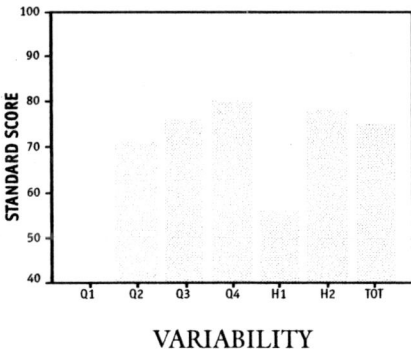

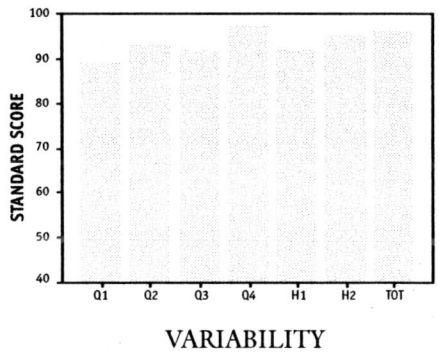

VARIABILITY   VARIABILITY

The variability score is considered to be a measure of inconsistency. Children with ADD are inconsistent – they can perform within normal limits for some of the time but then 'lose' it. This is considered to be the most measure of the TOVA test. Sam's post-test scores show a level of consistency that was not evident in his pre-test scores.

Although presented as an individual case study, Sam's progress is by no means unique and as more children come through the Clinic there are definite patterns emerging. Without exception every child has tested positive for milk intolerance and for many this has also included wheat and egg intolerances. All children have indicated problems with mineral levels and mineral imbalances. Sam's case and the others coming through the Clinic provide further support for the already growing volume of research linking nutrition and behaviour.

The Caregivers programme

The Caregivers Skills programme is a behavioural programme that works with parents and children with the objective of bringing about a change in the child's behaviour. This programme is based upon the work of David Stein (1999) who identified five stages necessary for bringing about change in a child's behaviour.

Stop the Drugs to Allow the Training of New Behaviours

Drugs control behaviour, but they also serve to mask the problem behaviours and thus block the way for effective change. The behaviours must be occurring if they are to be changed.

Treat Them as Normal and Capable Children

Attention disorders in this behavioural model are not diseases but patterns of inappropriate behaviours, faulty thinking, and lack of motivation. So-called ADD and ADHD children can be viewed as normal, but ones in whom the motivation to learn and perform well in school has failed to take hold and who have learned to behave in obnoxious ways. They are often lacking in consistency. Because neither ADD nor ADHD exists as a medical condition, the terminology for this program is changed. Children are referred to as inattentive (IA) and highly misbehaving (HM). The solution to eliminating IA and HM patterns is to teach parents and professionals the requisite skills to produce the desired changes.

Change the Way They Think as Well as the Way They Behave

The focal point of the Caregivers' Skills Program is to understand that IA and HM children have the classic mental state or cognitive thought pattern of 'not thinking'. This is a fundamental principle of Stein's approach and is why it works so well and why other programs collapse. Other traditional and typical approaches recommend a standard package of special tutoring, individual attention, medication, a few behaviour modification ideas, and perhaps a token economy program at home and at school. These methods actually reinforce and perpetuate the not-thinking pattern. Parents, teachers, and tutors constantly stay close to the child- prompting, guiding, cueing, coaxing, pointing things out, reminding, and warning. The adults do all the thinking for the child, who becomes highly dependent on assistance from other people. Adults become the child's reminder machines. The child does not learn the most basic, fundamental components necessary for obliterating the IA and HM (ADD and ADHD) patterns-namely, to focus, remember, pay attention, and monitor his/her own behaviour. This programme does not want mere compliance to what the adult is requesting but aims to teach the child to think and remember on his/her own.

Change Your Parenting

Every topic in this programme reverses much of what other approaches advocate. The Caregivers' Skills Programme teaches children to think and monitor their behaviours at all times, on their own, and with as little reminding and cueing as possible.

Change All Misbehaviours, Not Just the Behaviours of Impulsivity or Not Paying Attention

The Caregivers' Skills Program focuses on every behavioural and motivational problem, including aggression that may occur both in the home and at school. It teaches parents exactly what behaviours and thinking patterns are producing IA or HM problems and how to correct them.

The three programmes offered by the Clinic provide a more holistic approach to the management of children labelled with ADHD.

The research element of the Clinic reflects the need for evidence-based practice. If the medical model of treatment is to be challenged then it is incumbent upon advocates of alternative approaches to provide the evidence that these approaches are effective. It is also becoming clear that an integrative approach to the treatment of ADHD is necessary. For example, for those that have been medicated with Ritalin, Concerta or Strattera, there is evidence to suggest that, whilst it may help with focus and hyperactivity, it creates a condition of hyper focus. This means that a child may be able to read the words but has little comprehension of what is being read. (Woodhouse et al, 2004) Thus, whilst medication may have some effect on the behavioural aspect associated with ADHD, it does have a detrimental effect on academic achievement for the majority of children.

Many children experience problems in school because they have been given the diagnosis of ADHD and their behaviour may have caused problems. It is just as likely that their attention problem may have a cognitive cause and may be linked to a processing or a memory problem or a combination of cognitive problems. Consequently, because they cannot follow what is happening in the school situation, they become behavioural problems. Often this behaviour is regarded as symptomatic of ADHD. Whilst the above programmes may help in terms of behavioural issues they will not necessarily address the academic issues that were a precursor or consequence of the diagnosis of ADHD. Accordingly, the research component of the Clinic is also investigating a cognitive approach to dealing with ADHD. In this approach a full psychological profile of the child is obtained by the use of standardised psychological tests covering intelligence, mathematical and language ability, memory, processing speed and the ability to sustain attention on a specific task. Based on the profile, an individual educational programme is developed for each child to work through. Special curriculum materials are used that focus on a child's areas of under-development. An essential feature of the programme is that a child's maximum 'window' of attention is used as a means of moving from one task to another. If a child has an attention span of ten minutes then it is pointless setting tasks that go over that attention limit initially but with practice and over time this window can be increased. This work is based on the programme developed by Paul Cates in the USA with children diagnosed with ADHD. This programme has attained a high success rate in terms of helping children achieve in an academic situation. (Cates, 2004)

Summary

The work of the Clinic is still in its early days. It has yet to receive any support from the NHS who has ignored the research evidence that has accumulated over recent years and insist on seeing evidence of effectiveness solely on children coming through the Clinic. Therefore, those children being treated are either supported by some research funds or by the endowment fund set up by Steve Baldwin's family or are self-funding. There is mounting evidence that the programmes are effective in changing behaviour without any of the side effects that accompany a medication management programme for ADHD.

Conclusions and recommendations

To date it would appear that a majority of an unknown number of children are being treated for a disorder that we have little agreement as to its aetiology, with a medication of unknown pharmaco-physiological mechanisms although we do know that it has the potential for serious side-effects, both in the immediate and long-term situation, and that it has also been responsible for a number of deaths. If there are to be changes then there is a need for:

a) More of the medical profession to fully implement the NICE guidelines that call for a full diagnostic assessment of individual to include tests for possible co morbid conditions.

b) More medical and health professionals to be prepared to consider alternative approaches to the treatment of ADHD and other mental 'disorders'.

References

Arnold, L.E., Pinkham, S.M. and Votolato, N. (2000) Does zinc moderate essential fatty Acid and amphetamine treatment of ADHD. *Journal of Child and Adolescent Psychopharmacology* 10, 111-117.

Baldwin, S. (2000a) The cult of methylphenidate: clinical update. *Critical Public Health* 10, 81-86.

Baldwin, S. (2000b) Living in Britain: why are so many amphetamines prescribed to infants, children and teenagers in Britain? *Critical Public Health* 10, 451-462.

Biederman, J., Spencer, T. and Wilens, T. (2004) Evidence-based pharmacotherapy for attention-deficit hyperactivity disorder. *International Journal of Neuropsychopharmacology* 7, 77-97.

Burgess, J.R., Stevens, L., Wen Zhang, and Peck, L. (2000) Long-chain polyunsaturated fatty acids in children with attention-deficit hyperactivity disorder· *American Journal of Clinical Nutrition* 71, 327-320.

Buitelaar, J.K., Van der Gaag, R.J., Swaab-Barneveld, H. and Kuiper, M. (1995). Prediction of clinical response to methylphenidate in children with attention-deficit hyperactivity disorder. *Journal of the American Academy for Child and Adolescent Psychiatry* 34, 1025-32.

Cates, P. (2004) *Faith Christian Ministries.* Tennessee: USA

Crawford, M.A. (2000) The placental delivery of arachidonic and docosahexaenoic acids: implications for the lipid nutrition of the preterm infant. *American Journal of Clinical Nutrition* 71, S275-84.

Cushman, T., and Thomas, B. (2001) Understanding "inattention" in children and adolescents. *Ethical Human Sciences & Services* 3, 107-125.

Dommisse, J.V. (2000) Nutritional and other natural medical treatments for attention-deficit/hyperactivity disorder – AD(H)D. *Social Science Information Sur Les Sciences Sociales* 39, 489-504.

DuPaul, G.J., Barkley, R. A. and McMurray, M.B. (1994) Response of children with ADHD to methylphenidate: interaction with internalizing symptoms. *Journal of the American Academy for Child and Adolescent Psychiatry* 33, 894-903.

Evans L. (1999) Learning difficulties and nutrition: Pills or pedagogy? *Early Child Development & Care* 158, 107-111.

Ghoira, W. (2003) Investigation of information offered parents of ADD or ADHD elementary school students in San Diego county schools (California). *Dissertation Abstracts International.* Volume 64(1-A), 34, US: University Microfilms International.

Harding, K.L., Judah, R.D., Gant, C. (2003) Outcome-based comparison of Ritalin versus food-supplement treated children with AD/HD. *Alternative Medicine Review* 8, 319-30

Holman, R.T. (1998) The slow discovery of the importance of omega-3 essential fatty acids in human health. *Journal of Nutrition* 128, S427-33.

Holford, P. (1997) *The Optimum Nutrition Bible.* London: Piatkus Ltd.

Holford, P. (2003) *Optimum Nutrition for the Mind*. London: Piatkus Ltd.

Kidd, P.M. (2003) An approach to the nutritional management of autism. *Alternative Therapeutic Health* 9, 22-31.

NIH Consensus Statement. (1998). *Diagnosis and Treatment of Attention Deficit Hyperactivity Disorder (ADHD)*. National Institutes of Health, Bethesda.

Rasmussen, P. and Gillberg, C.J. (2000) Natural outcome of ADHD with developmental coordination disorder at age 22 years: a controlled, longitudinal, community-based study. *Journal of the American Academy for Child and Adolescent Psychiatry* 39, 1424-31.

Richardson, A.J. and Puri, B.K. (2002) A randomised double blind, placebo-controlled study of the effects of supplementation with highly unsaturated fatty acids on ADHD-related symptoms in children with specific learning difficulties. *Programmes in Neuropsychopharmacology and Biological Psychiatry* 26, 233-9.

Ross, B.M., McKenzie, I., Glen, I. and Bennett, C.P. (2003) Increased levels of ethane, a non-invasive marker of n-3 fatty acid oxidation, in breath of children with attention deficit hyperactivity disorder. *Nutritional Neuroscience* 6, 277-81.

Schnoll, R., Burshteyn, D., Cea-Aravena, J. (2003) Nutrition in the treatment of attention-deficit hyperactivity disorder: A neglected but important aspect. *Applied Psychophysiology And Biofeedback* 28, 63-75.

Shannon, S. (Ed). (2002). *Handbook of Complementary and Alternative Therapies in Mental Health*. (pp. 93-113). San Diego: Academic Press.

Steele, J. (2000) Exploring the relationship between diet and attention deficit hyperactivity disorder: The structure of nutritional intake of children with AD/HD as compared to normal controls. *Dissertation Abstracts International*. Vol 61(1-A), Jul, 87, US: University Microfilms International.

Stevens, L., et al (2003) EFA supplementation in children with inattention, hyperactivity, and other disruptive behaviours. *Lipids* 36, 1007-1021.

Stein, D., (1999) A medication-free parent management programme for children diagnosed with ADHD. *Ethical Human Sciences and Services* 1, 61-79.

Stordy, B.J. (2000) Dark adaptation, motor skills, docosahexaenoic acid and dyslexia. *American Journal of Clinical Nutrition* 71(Supp 1) 323S-326S.

Woodhouse D.J., Cates P., & Cates K. (2004) An On-going study on Psycho-Stimulants and the Cognitive Development of Children With ADHD. *American Neuropsychiatric Conference*. Bal Harbour Florida: Feb. 21

12
New Directions

Sami Timimi · Begum Maitra

The theme of this book is that child and adolescent psychiatry as a profession needs to develop a body of theory, and consequently practice, that is capable of making a much wider trawl of the literature, develop an ongoing dialogue with perspectives from other disciplines, and encourage an inclusion of ideas from other psychologies, other systems of medicine and other ways of practice, not just locally within our own culture but globally with cultures from other parts of the world and practices from other parts of the world.

We are aware that there is a professional culture that is afraid of taking risks, and that promotes a 'defensive' stance in the face of questioning and calls for change. This culture, though modulated to some extent by the recent, and very welcome, introduction of critical appraisal of the profession (more than of its belief systems), is kept in place by the opinion of a relatively small number of powerful academics (usually championing a biomedical orientation) whose theories fail to incorporate the evidence from contemporary clinical practice, and from alternative and equally respectable academic and research traditions within the social sciences. An example of how this conservatism undermines attempts to review practise is seen in the guidelines periodically produced by the National Institute of Clinical Excellence (NICE) in the UK. The approach, being hampered by the same view of what is acceptable research or evidence, fails to make a sufficiently radical analysis of the assumptions underlying existing theory and practice, or to take into account the wider body of data that is available and relevant. While, often helpfully, curbing some of the more extreme variations in clinical practice (such as the prescribing excesses), the guidelines amount to a homogenised version of professional constructs (such as of ADHD or childhood depression), unsupported by evidence, without questioning its premises, addressing controversies, and failing to make any substantive recommendations. The result, somewhat unsurprisingly, is a set of rather predictable, banal, and unnecessarily concrete guidelines that constrain rather than inform or facilitate responsive practice. While showing some ways in which clinicians might take a fresh look at their practice this book also asks how we might encourage others to explore what lies before them, and to question current professional dogma about its meanings and implications. We would like to be freer to discuss new ideas openly, to be supported in researching these, and to share in a genuine partnership with those we hope to treat since we rely wholly on their generosity and cooperation for material to understand the realities of children's lives, and on which we might build theoretical principles and therapeutic insights.

While much effort is being expended currently on finding some way to measure the 'outcomes' of current practice there seems little to suggest that we significantly alter the course of the bulk of what we call childhood 'disorders' in the West. We are certainly far from able to put together what we (claim to) know about contributory factors to protect children from the adverse experiences they suffer even within the relative affluence of the UK, and within the alleged protections offered by the welfare state. Child psychiatry theory and practice based on a set of rules that are considered universally valid, and applicable to any situation in order to discover a universal set of disorders, and their standardised treatments, is a dream that is evidently running thin, and is simply 'not delivering the goods'. We would like to see child and adolescent psychiatry, psychology and the allied therapeutic disciplines widen their theoretical scope so as to include the social, political, cultural and psychological realities that are essential to any consideration of health, and vitally, for an understanding of what is referred to under the rubric of 'mental health'. Here we come across a real problem with language, and especially in how languages (and cultures) arbitrarily separate realms of experience, the 'mental' from the 'physical', 'inner' from 'outer' (and the 'deep' from the 'superficial'). How might we use the multiplicity of cultural models available today inform a fresh way of considering the relationships between emotion, relationships and well-being, and ways of talking about these without an over-reliance on simple dichotomous categories? We would like to shift the paradigm from the modernist one of concrete 'facts' (such as 'risks' or 'disorders') that shade imperceptibly (and inevitably) into moral certainties, fostering the increasingly coercive therapeutic stance prevalent today, moving it towards the post-modern acknowledgement of relative and shifting meanings, and of the therapeutic potential contained in an enormous variety of verbal and non-verbal strategies, individual and collective, and limited only by imagination and the availability of supportive relationships.

The available evidence does not back the current mainstream dogma. More than that, we believe that the position we suggest is fundamentally more humane. Progressive clinical practice based on this more reflective position that we are advocating, listens to the dilemmas that the children and families face, engages them in a human dialogue and does not look for the approach easiest for the clinician by attributing meaning prematurely (as in diagnosing) and prescribing treatment (such as medication) that is least demanding of her/him (such as those placed by the role of therapist). While the efficacy of non-pharmacological treatments remains difficult to prove to the satisfaction of those who demand the supposed 'gold standard' of proof (namely, that provided by the randomised controlled trial) this approach, at the very least, protects patients from the substantial risks due to the side effects of medication. We remain convinced that in the absence of a body of evidence that shows better overall outcomes for conventional practice that the admittedly less conventional approaches this book points to are likely to be equally valid, and much more humane.

A summary of the recommendations from the chapters in this book

1   In Chapter 2 Jon Jureidini and Peter Mansfield argue that a more critical approach to ensuring the validity of published data on drug trails of psychiatric drugs used in childhood, is required in order to gain an adequate view of the benefits and harms of any given drug treatment. All drug trials should be registered at the time of their implementation and the details of those trials must be made available to major medical journals, so that when the papers are submitted, editors have the opportunity to assess the reported data against the aims set out in the initial protocol and any other as yet unpublished studies. They also advocate combining the knowledge that comes from Randomised Control Trials (RCTs) with pharmacoepidemiological data from observational studies, in order to gain an adequate view of the benefits and harms of any drug treatment. They also believe that antidepressant drugs cannot confidently be recommended as a treatment option for childhood depression.

2   In chapter 3 Begum Maitra claims that both alertness and humility are needed, if the professional disciplines are to base their claims of expertise on data that is not effectively obsolete, and dangerous to those whom they serve. Whilst the continuing demand for expertise in the 'health' arena is likely to remain, fuelled by its value as a major political counter, which professions will determine definitions of expertise and policy is likely to continue to change. It is especially important to be wary of the temptation to make unjustifiable claims for the mental health disciplines inspired by a political climate of endless 'innovation', and to periodically weigh up the validity and impact of our intrusions into private relationships. Begum Maitra cautions against over-reliance on professional relationships for the ordinary losses, hurts and grievances that life necessarily brings. In a climate of ambivalent regard for expertise, it is essential for mental health professionals to revitalise their fields, to abandon traditional islands of authority and enter fully into the richness of inter-disciplinary debate, research and a re-examination of the validity of its constructs.

3   In chapter 4 Rajeev Banhatti, Kedar Dwivedi and Begum Maitra using Indian culture as an example, show that the way childhood is conceptualised

in one culture (or subculture) has potentially far reaching and complex implications for a child's development. The goals of child development are influenced by how a culture constructs the meaning and purpose of life. They point out that traditional Indian conceptualisation of childhood and parenting appears to stress the holistic and integrative aspects of the relationship between man and nature, body and mind. Such a value system, they say, can lead to acceptance of imperfection, disease and misfortune, and to a culturally consonant form of resilience to adversity. The rapid and increasing exposure to global influences may expose children and young people (whether living in India or growing up outside it) to conflict between contradictory value systems, giving rise to hybrid cultural forms. These situations reveal both the pain and vulnerability created by rapid cultural change and the innovative strategies individuals create by re-interpreting cultural solutions. A useful orientation to cultural diversity would see it as a resource, of solutions devised over centuries to address human dilemmas in a wide variety of social and environmental contexts. The hierarchical positions allocated to 'modern' societies (or cultures, over 'traditional' ones) cause insidious damage to individuals in both. Cross-cultural practice requires that professionals maintain an attitude of curiosity leavened with humility when faced with other worldviews, beliefs and value systems.

4   In chapter 5 Charles Whitfield argues that there is strong evidence to suggest a link between a history of childhood trauma/abuse and subsequent behaviour problems including ADHD and violence/aggression. He points out that in these circumstances what appears to be the least expensive approach to managing a young child's behaviour (i.e. medication) may end up, in the long run, being the most costly. He recommends that children who present with behavioural symptoms, problems or disorders should be carefully screened and followed for a history of past and/or present childhood trauma. He asks how helpful is it to label children with new 'disorders' such as 'ADHD' when, instead, the child's behaviour may be a normal reaction to a difficult/stressful environment that they may find themselves in. He argues that by making these connections and offering treatment or an appropriate referral for protection, we can assist in all levels of prevention.

5   Jonathan Leo in chapter 6 believes that many of the studies on using psychotropic medication with children and adolescents appear to be written with at least one major goal being the development of a marketing plan. It is virtually impossible to dissect these studies and know where to draw the line between 'science' and 'marketing'. He feels that there are many proposals for solutions to the problem, but the single best way to prevent

this from happening is for doctors to pay more attention to the primary literature, and to place less reliance on second-hand sources. He says that we need to take a healthy dose of scepticism before reading pharmaceutical company brochures or when attending talks by pharmaceutical representatives, but it is now also evident that those doses of scepticism need to be taken, or maybe even increased, when reading medical journals. Doctors do not prescribe these medications just because pharmaceutical salespeople said childhood distress was a disease; they prescribed them because experts at medical schools writing in medical journals said it was a disease. He calls for a dose of common sense to enter the discussion. Of course children suffer, and they sometimes need help, but the medical community has become so enamoured with marketing, that it has ignored monumental shortcomings in the research that claims childhood distress are the result of disease states that require medication.

6   Having reviewed the history of the 'institutional' child to demonstrate that our institutional response to childhood deviance reflects the historical and cultural context of the time, Sami Timimi and Elisse Moody (chapter 7) conclude that current practice in adolescent in-patient units must also be considered as being historically and culturally embedded and likely to change as our ideas about the nature and cause of problematic behaviours, that we feel require institutional treatment, change. They provide an example from a UK adolescent in-patient unit, where they have developed a diagnosis free and virtually medication free environment, to demonstrate that alternatives to the current dominant construction used in most UK (and many other Western countries) adolescent mental health in-patient units (the medical model), is possible despite all the systemic constraints against this. Furthermore, they argue that the importance of challenging the hegemony of medicalisation is not only to demonstrate that positive outcomes can and do occur without reliance on the medical model, but also for showing that even those psychiatry would consider the most 'ill' can be helped in a way that provides a greater sense of hope for a young person's future than the idea of a fixed internal disease provides.

7   Eia Asen (chapter 8) suggests that clinicians need to be continuously looking to make and create relevant contexts that bring out the resourcefulness in families and help them to help themselves. The expertise of Child and Adolescent Mental Health Service (CAMHS) professionals' needs to shift from clinic based medically inspired practice to home and community based interventions, enabling families to connect with other families, rather than remaining over-connected with the helping system. This requires courage and innovative practices, including multiple service-user involvement, not as a politically imposed tokenism but as lived practice. Multiple family work,

involving 6 – 8 families sharing similar problems, could be developed in clinics as well as in schools and other settings. In this model the role of CAMHS clinicians changes to that of multi-modal workers, thus avoiding multiplication of helpers, as they are able – for a confined time – to deliver all the required interventions. Therapeutic intervention could then begin during the first encounter between family and clinician, as part of what might be termed a 'therapeutic assessment'. The related activities of context reading, context making and context managing could become essential skills that every CAMHS clinician possesses. In addition Eia Asen suggests that healthy irreverence towards any dogma, including the systemic one, is a prerequisite for good clinical practice and for respectful work with children, teenagers and their families.

8   In chapter 9 Sami Timimi proposes that in order to offer a holistic, integrated, multi-perspective model to help children who could be diagnosed with ADHD and their families, one first has to reject the notion that ADHD as label has anything meaningful or useful to offer clinical practice. He notes that paradoxically, although the use of the ADHD diagnosis and stimulant medication may appear to offer a cheap, labour saving way of helping children and their families, as with stimulants effectiveness it does the opposite. Although you may get quick results in the short term, in the long term you create a group of children who are dependent (on the drugs and the doctors who prescribe them) and need to carry on seeing their doctor for years (some say the rest of their lives), without, in many cases, ever having dealt with the original difficulties that led to help seeking. Sami Timimi sees his role as that of empowering children, parents and schools to find their own solutions so that dependency on doctors doesn't happen and clients can be discharged from clinics in a comparatively short time and with, he believes, at least as good an outcome (particularly in terms of client's satisfaction) than going down the more labour intensive (in the long term) diagnosis and medication route. He suggests a mixture of 'modernist' and 'post-modernist' approaches that can be used to help this client group without the need for medication.

9   In chapter 10 Sami Timimi in his critique of the notion of 'childhood depression' believes that medical researchers need to develop a more creative dialogue with researchers from other disciplines (such as sociology) to integrate within-body perspectives with broader ones. He argues that childhood depression is an individualised, context-depleted label that offers little explanatory power and can marginalize more helpful, context-rich explanations. He believes that the diagnosis of 'childhood depression' may first need to be abandoned before more comprehensive theory and

practice with regards to children's unhappiness can emerge. Having practiced without needing to diagnose anyone with 'childhood depression' or prescribe antidepressants to under eighteens for many years, he believes that abandoning the diagnosis offers a more humane and user friendly way of working than the easy option of giving a prescription when faced by emotional distress.

10 In chapter 11 David Woodhouse concludes that a large but unknown number of children are being treated for a disorder (ADHD) that we have little agreement as to its aetiology, with a medication of unknown pharmacophysiological mechanisms, that we know has the potential for serious side-effects, and that has been responsible for a number of deaths. If there are to be changes then there is a need for alternatives to medication to be offered, used and researched. He believes that more of the medical profession should fully implement the NICE guidelines that call for a full diagnostic assessment of the individual to include tests for possible co morbid conditions before diagnosing ADHD and prescribing medication. He calls for more medical and health professionals to be prepared to consider alternative approaches, to the treatment of ADHD, such as those used at the Cactus Clinic which includes nutritional and behavioural interventions.